Power, Privilege, and Public Health in the United States

Power, Privilege, and Public Health in the United States

Theory and Practice

Edited by
Lorraine T. Dean
Keilah A. Jacques

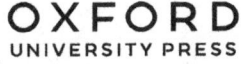

OXFORD
UNIVERSITY PRESS

OXFORD
UNIVERSITY PRESS

Oxford University Press is a department of the University of Oxford.
It furthers the University's objective of excellence in research, scholarship,
and education by publishing worldwide. Oxford is a registered trade mark of
Oxford University Press in the UK and in certain other countries.

Published in the United States of America by Oxford University Press
198 Madison Avenue, New York, NY 10016, United States of America.

Library of Congress Cataloging-in-Publication Data
Names: Dean, Lori, editor. | Jacques, Keilah A., editor.
Title: Power, privilege, and public health in the United States /
Lori Dean, Keilah Jacques. Description: New York, NY : Oxford University Press, [2024] |
Includes bibliographical references and index.
Identifiers: LCCN 2024056062 (print) | LCCN 2024056063 (ebook) | ISBN 9780197760925 (paperback) |
ISBN 9780197760949 (epub) | ISBN 9780197760956
Subjects: LCSH: Health services accessibility—United States. |
Discrimination in medical care—United States. | Social status—Health Aspects—United States. |
Equality—Health aspects—United States. | Public health—United States.
Classification: LCC RA418.3.U6 P66 2024 (print) | LCC RA418.3.U6 (ebook) |
DDC 362.10973–dc23/eng/20241226
LC record available at https://lccn.loc.gov/2024056062
LC ebook record available at https://lccn.loc.gov/2024056063

DOI: 10.1093/9780197760956.001.0001

Printed by Integrated Books International, United States of America

Contents

List of Figures

List of Tables

Preface

Lorraine T. Dean and Keilah A. Jacques

When I, Lori Dean, first started my faculty role at Johns Hopkins University in 2016, I learned that over 70% of Hopkins students were from families in the top 20% of the income distribution in the United States (*New York Times* 2017). As a faculty member at a school of public health with a stated goal to improve health around the world, especially those who are underserved, I wondered how we can equip students with the most privilege to serve those with the least privilege. This question doesn't just apply to trainees at elite academic institutions like Johns Hopkins: it applies to trainees of all post-secondary schools. Especially given that fewer than 15% of people in the US have a graduate degree (US Census Bureau 2022), anyone in higher education operates as part of a system of privilege (albeit not all at the same levels of privilege).

Privilege refers to a system of unearned advantages that reflect systems of economic and social oppression, which can have implications for health. Yet in trying to find materials to help students consider how their own level of privilege influenced the type of health questions they would answer as researchers, or the types of health challenges they would be assigned to solve as health practitioners, there were few resources. Further, the field of public health failed to confront the ways in which it was complicit in discriminatory structures that actually perpetuated poor health outcomes and health disparities throughout history. Given this gap in our curriculum, and a dearth of materials in academia, Keilah Jacques and I teamed up to develop a service-learning course titled "Methods for Assessing Power, Privilege, and Public Health in the United States." In 2019, our course was nationally recognized at the American Public Health Association's annual conference (our field's signature professional society event, with over 10,000 attendees) with the Delta Omega Award for Innovative Public Health Curriculum.

The success of our course may be attributed to the lack of materials for teaching these concepts in public health and medicine, even though many of these concepts have public health ramifications. Medical, nursing, and public health schools repeatedly cite a lack of resources for teaching about these concepts (Coleman 2020; Hagopian et al. 2018; Nairn et al. 2004; Ona et al. 2020;

Ufomata et al. 2021). In October 2023, the Council on Education for Public Health (CEPH), the accrediting body for public health programs, agreed to add a competency reflecting diversity, equity, and inclusion, after which there will need to be curricular resources available.

There is already demonstrated demand; for example, the successes of public health texts addressing racial privilege, including a recent "first" book led by Dr. Chandra Ford and published by the APHA (American Public Health Association) Press on racism and health that has sold out repeatedly since its introduction. Isabel Wilkerson's book about social class privilege, *Caste: The Origins of Our Discontents* was nominated for a national book award and has been a bestseller. The APHA and the Society of Behavioral Medicine have published statements denouncing racism and acknowledging privilege structures as a culprit, and over fifty-six top medical institutions issued similar statements in 2020 (Kiang and Tsai 2020). Both the Association of American Medical Colleges (AAMC) and the US-based Association for Prevention Teaching and Research (APTR) are designing antiracism toolkits to teach medical professionals (Papineni et al. 2021). We have witnessed the demand firsthand: a response to a June 2020 personal tweet about the Power, Privilege and Public Health course content garnered 175,000 impressions, 5,000 engagements, and nearly 2,000 link clicks. We believe this suggests that the time is ripe to expound on these topics with this first-ever book on power, privilege, and public health.

Distinctive Features and Organization of the Book

In the development of this book, we paid attention to privilege and equity in several ways.

First, we considered how we could advance equity in the organization of the book. In the academic space, coedited books often involve in-kind contributions from coauthors who are unpaid, while the coordinating editors receive ongoing royalties. We recognize that sometimes this is because the profit margins for academic books can be low, as they speak to small audiences and markets, but we also felt it was important to ensure that a book on power and privilege "walked the walk." We disrupted the traditional model and requested that our publishers, Oxford University Press, also offer some compensation to authors who spent their time and energy to contribute a chapter, which they gladly agreed. While this did require additional work and negotiation on our part, it reflects the intentionality and commitment to go out of our way to disrupt inequitable structures, which is expected and required for this work.

Second, we wanted to ensure that the book reflected perspectives from a diverse range of author types. In addition to considering the racial/ethnic and gender identities of authors, we considered the intellectual diversity and even the types of institutions represented—including authors from both within and outside academia. We also relied on sources that are outside of academic publications.

Third, we were committed to using public health examples that affect various populations; however, we acknowledge that most of the examples in this book focus on anti-Black racism. Because of the unique history of chattel slavery in the United States, Black Americans have faced the most egregious forms of denigration and have been subject to an orchestrated set of systems, policies, practices, and social norms to oppress Black Americans. Because of the length of this history, Black Americans have the most well-documented accounts of oppression, making these accounts useful, plentiful, and powerful to draw and learn from. In recognition that privilege is intersectional, we further recognize that Black women have borne the brunt of society's challenges and remain the most challenged when it comes to issues of health (e.g., having the highest maternal mortality rates of all groups), socioeconomic, and other outcomes. We draw from Janelle Jones's 2020 framework of "Black Women Best"—that if we resolve the challenges faced by Black women, all people will benefit (J. Jones 2020). While her framework applies largely to economic justice, we also believe that policies and practices that would disproportionately benefit the health of Black women would serve to benefit all others along the privilege gradient. Expanding on that, if we develop antiracist and equitable frameworks to advance Black women's health, that sets a foundation for developing antioppression action to advance other marginalized groups in the US.

Despite our intentionality, we also reflect on the limitations of this book:

- In one book, we cannot comprehensively address all issues or all populations. For this reason, we hope that this becomes just the first in a series of books by us and by other authors.
- The book is designed for audiences who want to learn about teaching about topics of privilege and health, though we believe it can have application to learners at many levels. We see this goal as being an informative guide and a tool for reflection on pedagogy and curriculum design.
- Currently, this book is focused on the US and is only available in English, meaning the examples and content may not be accessible to everyone, in every language. We hope that the increased uptake and attention to

privilege that this book can bring may help spur additional resources to expand the audiences we can reach.

- We strove for representation of identity but may not have achieved that in every identity domain. This was not for a lack of trying: we sincerely tried to be thoughtful about the coauthorship composition, which was also subject to who was willing and available to make a contribution.
- We write from the perspectives of people educated in Western societies and at elite and predominantly White institutions. Even though we cannot now change where we were educated, we hope to use the privilege from these spaces in ways that better the health field and society, starting with the contribution of this book.

Acknowledgments

In the spirit of critical self-reflection, we acknowledge the role of life challenges, professional and personal disruptions, global events, and political affronts that compelled rest, grace, collaboration, and innovation as the power-with and power-within needed to bring this timely and foundational work to fruition.

We would like to acknowledge the many people who brought life to this book project:

Charlie Nguyen, for your help with editing and reference checking, and Dr. Dustin Duncan, who connected us to Oxford University Press, the publishers who have supported and championed this text. We honor the curricular contributions of Dr. Katrina Bell McDonald, whose lectures on power and privilege framed many of the definitions used in this book, and the Johns Hopkins graduate students whose independent study course was the prototype for what later became the power and privilege course that prompted the idea for this book: Dr. Abigail Greenleaf, Mara James, Dr. Jocelynn Owusu, Dr. Emily Knapp, Sally Safi, Dr. Kate Leifheit, Dr. Yousra Yusuf, Rachel Viqueira, and Anna Abelson. We thank mentors like Dr. Constance Lacy, who not only modeled education as liberation, but taught the pedagogy of power-sharing and privilege checking as a foundation for institutional change. We thank the many contributors to the course's success, including course TAs: Dr. Kate Leifheit, Eli Pousson, Dr. Ruoxi Yu, and Angela D'Adamo; and students who championed the course: Sevly Snguon and Dr. Mudia Uzzi. We thank the leadership at Johns Hopkins, especially members of the Department of Epidemiology (Dr. David Celentano, Laura Camarata, and Fran Burman), and the Johns Hopkins University SOURCE Office, who championed this course and provided resources toward its development and maintenance. We thank the local Baltimore community partners who taught us even more than a textbook could about how power and privilege have impacted our society and how it frames relationships between academic institutions and communities: Men and Families Center, Blue Water Baltimore, Center for Urban Families, and Community Law Center. We also extend thanks to our academic support circles who encouraged us through the creation of this book: Dr. Renee Johnson, Dr. Vanya Jones, Dr. Kassandra Alcaraz, and Dr. Chidinma Ibe. We honor that we wrote this book during times of deep grief in both of our lives and were not operating at our peak capacities; nevertheless, we hope this book makes an important and valuable contribution. We are grateful to our parents, grandparents, family members, and ancestors who loved us and inspired us through this process and whose legacies live on through us in the impact that this book will make.

References

Coleman, Tesiah. 2020. "Anti-Racism in Nursing Education: Recommendations for Racial Justice Praxis." *Journal of Nursing Education* 59 (11): 642–645.

Hagopian, Amy, Kathleen Mcglone West, India J. Ornelas, Ariel N. Hart, Jenn Hagedorn, and Clarence Spigner. 2018. "Adopting an Anti-Racism Public Health Curriculum Competency: The University of Washington Experience." *Public Health Reports* 133 (4): 507–513.

Jones, Janelle. 2020. "Black Women Best." Data for Progress, July 15, 2020. https://www.dataforprogress.org/blog/2020/7/15/black-women-best.

Kiang, Mathew V., and Alexander C. Tsai. 2020. "Statements Issued by Academic Medical Institutions after George Floyd's Killing by Police and Subsequent Unrest in the United States: Cross-Sectional Study." *medRxiv.* https://doi.org/10.1101/2020.06.22.20137844.

Nairn, Stuart, Carolyn Hardy, Logan Parumal, and Glenn A. Williams. 2004. "Multicultural or Anti-Racist Teaching in Nurse Education: A Critical Appraisal." *Nurse Education Today* 24 (3): 188–195.

New York Times. 2017. "Economic Diversity and Student Outcomes at Johns Hopkins." The Upshot, January 18, 2017. https://www.nytimes.com/interactive/projects/college-mobility/johns-hopkins-university.

Ona, Fernando F., Ndidiamaka N. Amutah-Onukagha, Rina Asemamaw, and Anthony L. Schlaff. 2020. "Struggles and Tensions in Antiracism Education in Medical School: Lessons Learned." *Academic Medicine: Journal of the Association of American Medical Colleges* 95 (12S): S163–S168.

Papineni, Padmasayee, Sarah Filson, Tiffanie Harrison, and Malachi McIntosh. "Adopting an Anti-Racist Medical Curriculum." 2021. The BMJ Opinion, February 19, 2021. https://blogs.bmj.com/bmj/2021/02/19/adopting-an-anti-racist-medical-curriculum/

Ufomata, Eloho, Sarah Merriam, Aditi Puri, Katherine Lupton, Darlene LeFrancois, Danielle Jones, Attila Nemeth, Laura K. Snydman, Rachel Stark, and Carla Spagnoletti. 2021. "A Policy Statement of the Society of General Internal Medicine on Tackling Racism in Medical Education: Reflections on the Past and a Call to Action for the Future." *Journal of General Internal Medicine* 36 (4): 1077–1081.

US Census Bureau. 2022. "Census Bureau Releases New Educational Attainment Data." February 24, 2022. https://www.census.gov/newsroom/press-releases/2022/educational-attainment.html.

List of Contributors

Lorraine T. Dean, ScD, is an associate professor, Department of Epidemiology, John Hopkins Bloomberg School of Public Health, Baltimore, MD, USA.

Keilah A. Jacques, LMSW, is an adjunct instructor, John Hopkins Bloomberg School of Public Health and School of Nursing, Baltimore, MD, USA.

anushka r. aqil, PhD, is an instructor at Johns Hopkins University, Baltimore, MD, USA.

Greta Bauer, PhD, MPH, is an adjunct research professor, Epidemiology and Biostatistics at Western University, London, Canada, and a professor and director, Eli Coleman Institute for Sexual and Gender Health at University of Minnesota, Minneapolis, MN, USA.

Lindsay Beavers, MPT, BSc.Kin, is an adjunct lecturer at Physical Therapy Department, Temerty Faculty of Medicine, University of Toronto, Toronto, Canada.

Chelsey R. Carter, PhD, MPH, is an assistant professor, Social and Behavioral Sciences at Yale University, New Haven, CT, USA.

Tekisha Dwan Everette, PhD, MPA, MPH, CPH, is an assistant professor adjunct at Yale School of Public Health, New Haven, CT, USA.

Sharon D. Jones-Eversley, DrPH, MA, BA, CNP, is Professor Emeritus at Department of Family Science, Towson University, Towson, MD, USA.

Gilbert C. Gee, PhD, is Professor and Chair in the Department of Community Health Sciences at Fielding School of Public Health at UCLA, Los Angeles, CA, USA.

Keon L. Gilbert, PhD is Professor in the College for Public Health and Social Justice at St. Louis University, St. Louis, MO, USA and fellow in the Governance Studies program at The Brookings Institution in Washington, DC, USA.

Darrell Hudson, PhD, MPH, is Professor and Chair in the Department of Health Behavior & Health Equity, University of Michigan, Ann Arbor, MI, USA.

Danya E. Keene, PhD, is an associate professor at Yale School of Public Health, New Haven, CT, USA.

Krystal O. Lee, MPA, EdD, is a research associate in the Department of Health, Behavior and Society at Johns Hopkins Univeristy Bloomberg School of Public Health, Baltimore, MD, USA.

Amelea Lowery, MPH, is a graduate student at Yale School of Public Health, Yale University, New Haven, MD, USA.

Graham Mooney, PhD, is an associate professor, Department of the History of Medicine at Johns Hopkins University, Baltimore, MD, USA.

Eric Cesar Morales, PhD, is the Resourcing Coordinator at Philly Thrive, Philadelphia, PA, USA.

Stephanie A. Nixon, PT, PhD, is Vice Dean, Faculty of Health Sciences, and Director, School of Rehabilitation Therapy at Queen's University, Kingston, Canada.

Angie Phenix, DSc(c), MEd, MOT, is an occupational therapist at Phenix OT Consulting, Regina, Saskatchewan, Canada.

Meredith Smith is an assistant professor, Teaching Stream at Department of Physical Therapy, University of Toronto, Canada, and a clinical teaching and learning educator at University Health Network, Toronto, Canada.

Sherrie Flynt Wallington, PhD, is an associate professor, Health Disparities & Oncology at George Washington University School of Nursing, Milken Institute School of Public Health, Washington, DC, USA.

Chapter 1
Introduction

Lorraine T. Dean and Keilah A. Jacques

Privilege refers to a system of unearned advantages that reflect systems of economic and social oppression, which can have significant implications for both an individual's health and the health of a community, state, or country (Davis and Harrison 2013). The science of teaching about privilege and health is in its nascency; however, scholarship on privilege has much deeper origins. Many begin teaching about privilege with Dr. Peggy McIntosh's foundational piece, "White Privilege: Unpacking the Invisible Knapsack" (McIntosh 1988). In that piece, Dr. McIntosh detailed how challenging it is for people who have the most privilege to recognize it while carrying it and using its tools daily. Her paper addressed male, White, and heterosexual privilege while also acknowledging the need to study privilege by age, ability, ethnicity, religion, and nationality. She highlighted the insidiousness of the invisibility of privilege and how the myopia around privilege precludes system-level changes that would be needed to have an equitable society. Her highly acclaimed and must-read piece put an academic spotlight on an issue that others before her had highlighted outside the academy.

For example, over 125 years before Dr. McIntosh's publication, in 1851, the formerly enslaved Black female activist Sojourner Truth issued her "Aint I a Woman" speech at the Ohio Women's Rights Convention, laying bare the intersections of privilege along axes of gender and race that continued to hinder her ability to have full rights in society (Sojourner Truth 1851). The concept of intersectionality was introduced by bell hooks (Hooks 1984) and Dr. Kimberlé Crenshaw (Crenshaw 2013) contemporarily with Dr. McIntosh's piece to show that an individual's membership in marginalized groups defined by race, gender, class, sexual identity, religion, ability, and nationality intersect in ways that lead to a complex profile of privilege for each person. In public health, we still have yet to define methods that can help fully capture how these complex profiles of identity contribute to health disparities, though

Lorraine T. Dean and Keilah A. Jacques, *Introduction*. In: *Power, Privilege, and Public Health in the United States.* Edited by: Lorraine T. Dean and Keilah A. Jacques, Oxford University Press. © Oxford University Press (2025). DOI: 10.1093/9780197760956.003.0001 scholars like Dr. Greta Bauer, Dr. John Jackson, and Dr. Ayden Scheim have made methodological advances in that area.[1]

As evidenced by a PubMed search on "privilege" and terms related to race, sex or gender, religion, immigration status, neurodivergence, and language, the past ten years have seen substantial growth in both empirical and nonempirical peer-reviewed contributions on the topic of teaching about privilege. Still, as can be seen in Figure 1.1, the overall number of papers is small: thirty-one empirical papers, eighteen of which were intervention studies around testing elements of curriculum and twenty-five nonempirical commentary or reflection pieces.

Most of the intervention studies have involved brief training of nine hours or less and found statistically significant or qualitatively different changes in how people viewed themselves or their knowledge and awareness of privilege and oppression structures (Alexander-Ruff and Kinion 2019; Borowsky, Morinis, and Garg 2021; Brown, White, and Gregory 2021; Chang et al. 2019; Chow, Case, and Matias 2019; Davis et al. 2021; Ellison et al. 2021; Herzog et al. 2021; Holdren et al. 2023; Holm et al. 2017; Jindal et al. 2022; Martinez et al. 2021; Siemers and Kenyon 2022; Witten and Maskarinec 2015; Wu et al. 2019; Zanders and Colquitt 2023; Alexander et al. 2024; Beavers et al. 2024; Brown and Jones 2024). Recent evidence suggests that even a single class session on privilege and health can change someone's perspective on

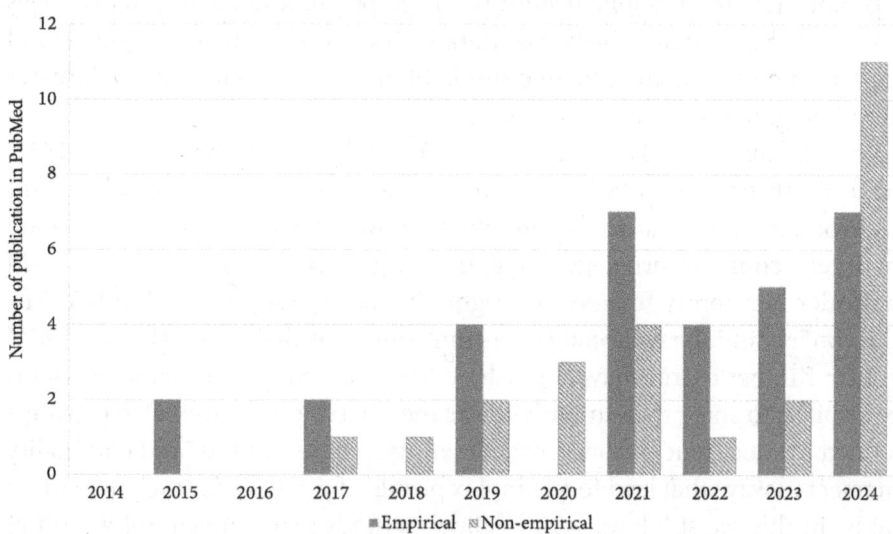

Figure 1.1 Publications on teachings about privilege and health in PubMed, January 1, 2014 to December 31, 2024.
Source: Conceptualized and designed by the authors.

[1] These scholars also acknowledge that the experience of intersectionality cannot fully be quantified and require other methods to understand it.

privilege (Witten and Maskarinec 2015), (imagine what an entire curriculum on these topics might do!) but there are literally no higher education academic book titles on privilege *and health* as a general topic.

How can instructors equip health-focused higher education students, who are among the most privileged, to serve those who are least privileged? While public health and medicine intend to heal individuals and communities in need, at times the unequal power and privilege of practitioners compared to the populations they serve have unintentionally done harm, and more must be done to ensure that future practitioners do not repeat the mistakes of the past. We offer this text as a tool to be used in teaching about theories of power and privilege (Chapters 2-7), with a specific lens for how scholars, clinicians, and practitioners in public health, medicine, and allied fields can apply this knowledge (Chapters 8-12).

Use of Terminology and Language

Throughout this book, we will refer to several key terms (Table 1.1), especially the ones in the title of the book: power and privilege. Other key terms will be defined within chapters, including "dominant group" (Chapter 2); "health disparities" and "health equity" (Chapter 4); "justice" (Chapter 10); "critical race theory" (Chapters 5 and 7); "intersectionality" (Chapter 6), and "scientific racism" and "racial capitalism" (Chapter 8); however, in this introductory section, we orient our readers to the terms defined below.

First, we start with **power**. Power is defined as the ability to influence, define, direct, and determine behavior as a result of having access to resources (Amenta, Andrews, and Caren 2018; Battilana and Casciaro 2021; Ladkin and Probert 2021). However, defining systems of power in relationship to health requires a consideration of the sociopolitical agreements or relationships between individuals and institutions and the ability of agents of power to direct the definitions, resources, opportunities, and pathways to health (Shawar et al. 2019). When power is leveraged, it is operated through **levers of power**, or "elements within political systems that individuals and groups can engage to influence or bring about change in the system or results ("Civic Knowledge Rubric," n.d.). In contrast, when power is abused, that is called **oppression**. Oppression is defined as "the systematic subjugation of one social group by a more powerful social group for the social, economic, and political benefit of the more powerful social group" (Delgado, & Jean 2023). Oppression requires four conditions: "(1) the oppressor group has the power to define reality for themselves and others, (2) the target groups take in and internalize the negative messages about them and end up cooperating with the oppressors (thinking and acting like them), (3) [oppression is] systematic and institutionalized, so that individuals are not necessary to keep it going, and (4) members of both the oppressor and target groups are socialized to play their roles as normal and correct" (Berman, Cohen, and Mills 2023; Collins, & Bilge 2020; Delgado, & Jean 2023; Morgan 1996). Oppression is not the same as **discrimination**, as discrimination can occur even at equal levels of the power gradient and is defined as biased actions based on a prejudice against an individual or group characterized by race, class, sexual orientation, age, disability, or other characteristic (Braveman 2014; Braveman & Gotman 2014).

Racism refers to a system of power and the consequent beliefs and actions based on a socially defined racial hierarchy where some groups are oppressed, marginalized, or denied resources based on their socially assigned racial grouping. (Williams, Lawrence, and Davis 2019). Racism can occur at multiple levels, including internalized, interpersonal (or personally mediated), institutional (Jones 2000), and structural (Dean and Thorpe 2022).

Structural racism is a particular form of oppression that speaks to "the totality of ways in which societies foster [racial] discrimination, via mutually reinforcing [inequitable] systems . . . (eg, in housing, education, employment, earnings, benefits, credit, media, health care, criminal justice, etc) that in turn reinforce discriminatory beliefs, values, and distribution of resources', reflected in history, culture, and interconnected institutions" (Bailey et al. 2017) (p. 1454). Unlike racism at other levels, including interpersonal and intrapersonal (Jones 2000), structural racism emphasizes how the *interconnectedness* of institutions, systems, norms, and beliefs produces racially inequitable structures and practices, even if the original design of those structures was not intentionally racist (Bailey et al. 2017; Dean and Thorpe 2022).

Here, we note that we reject race as a biological factor. Race reflects social and ideological conventions imposed by society, and racial/ethnic inequities in health are due to embodied racism. Despite some people's insistence on race as biological and an entire body of evidence rebutting them, the American Anthropological Society has clearly stated, "Evidence from the analysis of genetics (e.g., DNA) indicates that most physical variation, about 94%, lies within so-called racial groups. . . . This means that there is greater variation within 'racial' groups than between them. . . . any two individuals within a particular population are about as different genetically as any two people selected from any two populations in the world" (Bamshad et al. 2004; https://americananthro.org/about/policies/statement-on-race/). We also distinguish race from genetic ancestry, which is about exposures and selection over time that occurred to people and groups who lived in similar geographic areas or who shared languages, but we are careful not to conflate that with our social racial categories.

Next, we define **privilege**. Privilege refers to "unearned rights, benefits, immunity, and favors that are bestowed on individuals and groups only on the basis of their race, culture, religion, gender, sexual orientation, physical ability, or other key characteristics" (Davis and Harrison 2013). Privilege has two major components: unearned advantage, an unearned entitlement that is restricted to certain groups, and conferred dominance, or giving one group power over another because of their group membership. One does not necessarily have to be part of a traditionally privileged group to benefit from it. Privilege is assigned to people based on being perceived as part of a group that is privileged, but being identified as part of the privileged group does not mean that every individual in that group has power to exercise that privilege. Instead, it means that the people in that privileged group can identify that society values the characteristic that offers privilege, making it easier to access power than it is for groups who are not aligned with a privileged identity (Johnson 2005a, 2005b).

Sociologist Dr. Allen G. Johnson uses the example of male privilege in a male-dominated society; it does not mean that all people perceived to be males have power, but that "every man can identify with power as a value that his culture associates with manhood, and this identification makes it easier for any man to assume and use power in relation to others.... Since women are culturally *dis*identified with power, it's harder for them to exercise it in any situation. When women do find ways to be powerful, it's usually in spite of the male-dominated character of a patriarchal system as a whole" (p. 91). While Johnson uses male privilege as an example, this can be applied to privilege based on other characteristics as well.

Positionality refers to where someone is in the social hierarchy, based on the privilege gradient, and how that relates to how they interact with others on the gradient and view the world. Being a privileged group means that society caters to that group and sees that group as a "referent group," or default to which everyone else is compared. In the context of health, this might be reflected in health disparity studies that, for example, automatically use White as the referent group to which all other health is compared. This is problematic for several reasons.

First, it may be unrealistic to use a referent group that has benefitted from long-term societal privilege: using their health as a referent may result in using an "overprivileged standard" to which to benchmark health. While some people might say that we should use as our referent the group that has had the most societal advantages as a way to show what everyone's health could be like if they had the same advantages, it fails to acknowledge that what we perceive as good health may be a result of overuse and abuse of resources that may have diminishing returns. For example, several studies have shown that White adults in the US use more healthcare services than Black adults (Dickman et al. 2022), spend more on healthcare even when under the same insurance plans and at equal levels of health as Black adults, and spend a greater proportion on primary or specialty care than emergency department (ED) care (Dieleman et al. 2021; Dean et al. 2023). Thus, using healthcare expenditures for White people as a standard may be comparing an extreme that does not reflect a level of healthcare that is reasonably needed for optimal health.

Second, using the most privileged group as the referent fails to acknowledge that even groups not aligned with privilege can and do have positive health outcomes. For example, in studies of alcohol use disorder among US youth, Black youths may be the best referent, as Black youths have lower rates of alcohol use disorder than White youths. Using White youths as a default referent group bakes in a biased belief that White behavior and outcomes will always be the best or preferred.

Third, using the most privileged group as the referent presumes that their standard should be catered to, rather than the default or standard being something that is accessible to everyone. The antiableism community has called out design flaws that are not inclusive, such as websites that have no text enlargement feature for those who are visually impaired, and buildings that have no wheelchair ramps or that have narrow door frames and unpaved or uneven sidewalks. These are features that could benefit even people who do not identify as disabled, but even if these features did not have universal benefit, dismantling power and privilege structures means being open to "centering at the margins," or developing resources or systems that specifically cater to and target people who have been marginalized. The disability inclusion community has adopted the mantra "Nothing about us without us" to demand equal participation in decisions that can help ensure that the needs of differently abled persons are met.

What is also significant about the privilege standard is the unspoken role of power. Through the lens of power-over (as defined in Chapter 2), the ability to situate a group or a norm in place as the highest rung in the social hierarchy requires the ability to relationally establish the privilege gradient, let alone establish the norm of utilizing the gradient as the measuring stick for other social groups—having the ability to call this concept of privilege into question and reimagine what qualifiers and definitions of health can and should be.

These key concepts operate as part of the spectrum of privilege, which occur across different axes of identity. We use "privilege" as an umbrella term that encompasses the study of three major (nonexhaustive) domains: economic privilege (e.g., generational wealth and legacy benefits), social privilege (e.g., racial hierarchies, immigration status, and sexuality), and somatic privilege (e.g., phenotype, neuro-types, and ability status). The umbrella metaphor is intended to suggest that all identities fall along the spectrum of

Table 1.1 Key terms and definitions

Key term	Definition
Power	The ability to influence, define, direct, and determine behavior, as a result of having access to resources (Amenta et al. 2018; Battilana and Casciaro 2021; Ladkin and Probert 2021).
Levers of Power	Elements within political systems that individuals and groups can engage to influence or bring about change in the system or results ("Civic Knowledge Rubric," n.d.).
Oppression	"The systematic subjugation of one social group by a more powerful social group for the social, economic, and political benefit of the more powerful social group" (Hardiman 2007; Merriam-Webster, n.d.).
Privilege	Unearned rights, benefits, immunity, and favors that are bestowed on individuals and groups only on the basis of their race, culture, religion, gender, sexual orientation, physical ability, or other key characteristics (Davis and Harrison 2013).
Discrimination	Biased actions based on a prejudice against an individual or group characterized by race, class, sexual orientation, age, disability, or other characteristic (Davis and Harrison 2013; Adams et al. 2022).
Racism	A system of power and consequent beliefs and actions based on a socially defined racial hierarchy where some groups are oppressed, marginalized, or denied resources based on their socially assigned racial grouping. (Williams, Lawrence, and Davis 2019). Racism can occur at multiple levels, including internalized, interpersonal (or personally mediated), and institutional (Jones 2000).
Structural racism	"The totality of ways in which societies foster [racial] discrimination, via mutually reinforcing [inequitable] systems . . . (eg, in housing, education, employment, earnings, benefits, credit, media, health care, criminal justice, etc) that in turn reinforce discriminatory beliefs, values, and distribution of resources, reflected in history, culture, and interconnected institutions"(Bailey et al. 2017).
Positionality	The location of where someone is in the social hierarchy, based on the privilege gradient and how that relates to how they interact with others on the gradient and view the world. Being a privileged group means that society caters to that group, and sees that group as a "referent group," or default to which everyone else is compared (Carter and Legleitner 2021).
Resilience	The ability to build a practice of rest and restoration that supports becoming strong, healthy, or successful again after something happens. The ability of something, due to a significant margin, to return to its original shape after it has been pulled, stretched, bent, and so on. An ability to recover from or adjust easily to misfortune or change due to a well-supported nature (Brown 2017).

privilege: there is no one group that has access to all levels of privilege or any one group that has absolutely none; there is variation within groups, but we all are somewhere under the umbrella. The umbrella domains in Figure 1.2 highlight features by which groups are structurally oppressed; while individual people may also be discriminated against based on other features, the ones explicitly in the umbrella focus on groups with explicit structural oppressions. Further, studying privilege requires attention to power, positionality, resources, and even time (Gee et al. 2019).[2]

One of the key aspects of power and privilege is that they are explicit in naming their sources and roots. In the context of health, this means going beyond talking about the results of power and privilege gradients—that is, talking about the health inequities created by how power and privilege are levied. Instead, power and privilege constructs require that we identify who has or lacks power and how that confers elements of privilege. In the case of the US, White Supremacy Culture is at the root of several forms of oppression and should be explicitly named; White Supremacy Culture is defined in detail in Chapter 9, which cites ways in which it applies to examples of health. Of note, it does not require being White-bodied to be purveyors of White Supremacy Culture, as power and benefits may be conferred upon people of any race who endorse its tenets. For example, we as writers of this book reflect on our roles as two Black women who are also members of an elite, predominantly White-bodied institution steeped in White Supremacy Culture.

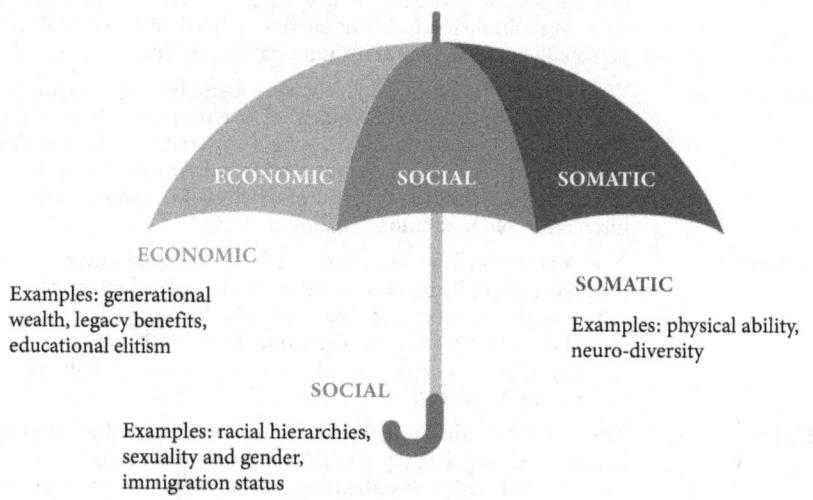

Figure 1.2 Umbrella diagram of domains of privilege.
Source: Figure conceptualized and designed by the authors; graphic provided by Template by PresentationGO [www.presentationgo.com]; terms and conditions apply [https://www.presentationgo.com/terms-conditions/].

[2] Dr. Gil Gee's paper highlights how time is differentially available and structured differently based on people's racial identity and access to racial privilege, such that, due to racism, Black people have less access to social or leisure time because of historic and current separation from resources and less biological time due to premature aging, weathering, and premature mortality.

Although our racial and gender identities align us with positions of low privilege and power, so long as we endorse the metrics of success defined by our institution that are informed by White Supremacy Culture—for example, overworking—we can experience some of the benefits of White Supremacy Culture while simultaneously being oppressed by it.

While much of this book focuses on the challenges of power and privilege and the oppression it can bring, we also lift up the *resilience* and *resistance* of groups who have been marginalized. We define "resilience" as the ability to build a practice of rest and restoration that supports becoming strong, healthy, or successful in spite of what happens. The ability of something, due to a significant margin, to return to its original shape after it has been pulled, stretched, bent, and so on is an ability to recover from or adjust easily to misfortune or change due to a well-supported nature (Brown 2017). We define "resistance" as the ability to cause or withstand disruption. We see the publication of this text in itself as a form of resilience and resistance and hope that it is the first of many texts that can help train health and medical trainees and professionals.

Another major theme of this book is the concept that the health of one group is often "traded off" for the health of another group. In an example shared by Dr. Sharon Jones-Eversley: consider the case of George Floyd, who was murdered by asphyxiation by police officers in 2020. When police arrived in response to a call that Floyd had used a counterfeit $20 bill to buy cigarettes, George Floyd was sober and not acting violently. Yet he was forcefully yanked from his car, handcuffed behind his back, and made to sit on the ground before police officer Derrick Chauvin knelt on his neck and chest for nine minutes and twenty-nine seconds until he took his last breath. The officers used plastic gloves to protect themselves from germs but did not extend health and humanity to Mr. Floyd. The literature on anti-Black structural racism includes several studies showing that the impact of structural racism on health is neutral or beneficial to White Americans while detrimental to the health of Black Americans (Dougherty et al. 2020; Lukachko et al. 2014; Wallace et al. 2017). We offer these as contemporary examples, and Chapter 11 expands on other examples cited in health literature.

We reject that trading one group's health for another group's health is necessary and believe that, especially in a place as resource-rich as the United States, there is sufficiency for everyone to have access to achieving a reasonable standard of health.

Finally, we note that this book is intended to demonstrate the need for critical self-reflection throughout the process of learning about teaching about power and privilege. These topics ask us to inspect ourselves, our biases, and our advantages, and continue to reflect and reinspect them through the dynamic changes to our lives and identities. This is especially important given the likelihood of emotional reactivity to teaching and learning about privilege. Dr. Eric Morales has highlighted some of the common ways in which reactivity (Morales 2020) to these topics may occur:

- Headwind/tailwind asymmetry, which reflects a bias in how people assess privileges and adversities in their lives. Much in the same way a cyclist might more easily recognize the headwind preventing them from moving forward on their bike but might overlook the tailwind pushing them forward, it is often easier for people to see the adversities preventing them from moving forward, while overlooking the privileges pushing them forward (Davidai and Gilovich 2016).
- Backfire effect, which reflects that when people are presented with facts that contradict their long-held beliefs or views (Nyhan and Reifler 2010), they may recoil and more firmly adhere to their original position as a defense strategy.

We see critical reflection as a way to stay grounded and to continue to center humaneness in the work of addressing power and privilege and to manage the resistance that we may feel in ourselves when confronted with our own privilege. Chapters 10, 11 and 12 use critical reflection to share insights on our reactions to how privilege teachings have been received in the academic courses we teach.

In total, this book brings together teachings from leading scholars on aspects of privilege and health. It is designed to give trainees and public health educators foundational knowledge on theories of power and privilege that can be used to understand health distributions, differences, and disparities. It offers practical guidance for developing antioppressive competencies and experiential self-reflective activities to examine how our own power and privilege influence the design and interpretation of health studies. We hope that this text becomes a pivotal point for greater scholarship, practice, and self-reflection that is attentive to how power and privilege impact health and medicine research, policy, and clinical practice.

References

Adams, Maurianne, Lee Anne Bell, Diane J. Goodman, Davey Shlasko, Rachel R. Briggs, and Romina Pacheco. 2022. *Teaching for Diversity and Social Justice*. New York: Routledge.

Alexander-Ruff, Julie H., and Elizabeth S. Kinion. 2019. "Developing a Cultural Immersion Service-Learning Experience for Undergraduate Nursing Students." *Journal of Nursing Education* 58 (2): 117–120.

Alexander, A.B., M. Palmer, D. Palmer, K. Pettit. 2024. "'Showing up to the Conversation': Qualitative Reflections from a Diversity, Equity, and Inclusion Book Club with Emergency Medicine Leadership." *Acad Emerg Med.* 10.1111/acem.15034.

Amenta, Edwin, Kenneth T. Andrews, and Neal Caren. 2018. "The Political Institutions, Processes, and Outcomes Movements Seek to Influence." In *The Wiley Blackwell Companion to Social Movements*, 447–465. Chichester, UK: John Wiley & Sons.

Bailey, Zinzi D., Nancy Krieger, Madina Agénor, Jasmine Graves, Natalia Linos, and Mary T. Bassett. 2017. "Structural Racism and Health Inequities in the USA: Evidence and Interventions." *Lancet* 389 (10077): 1453–1463.

Bamshad, Michael, Stephen Wooding, Benjamin A. Salisbury, and J. Claiborne Stephens. 2004. "Deconstructing the Relationship between Genetics and Race." *Nature Reviews Genetics* 5 (8): 598–609.

Battilana, Julie, and Tiziana Casciaro. 2021. *Power, for All: How It Really Works and Why It's Everyone's Business.* Simon and Schuster.

Beavers, L., T. Vo, J. Lee, T. Duvage, H. Mullins, A. Tewari, A. Needham, R. Brydges. 2024. "Using Virtual Reality Simulation to Address Racism in a Healthcare Setting." *Adv Simul (Lond)* 9 (1): 46. 10.1186/s41077-024-00322-2.

Berman, Stacie Brensilver, Robert Cohen, and Ryan Mills. 2023. "Why CRT Belongs in the Classroom, and How to Do It Right." *History News Network.* January 22, 2023. http://hnn.us/article/184803.

Borowsky, Hannah, Leora Morinis, and Megha Garg. 2021. "Disability and Ableism in Medicine: A Curriculum for Medical Students." *MedEdPORTAL: The Journal of Teaching and Learning Resources* 17 (January): 11073.

Brown, Adrienne M. 2017. *Emergent Strategy: Shaping Change, Changing Worlds.* AK Press.

Brown, Elizabeth A., Brandi M. White, and Aramis Gregory. 2021. "Approaches to Teaching Social Determinants of Health to Undergraduate Health Care Students." *Journal of Allied Health* 50 (1): e31–36.

Brown, E.A., R., Jones. 2024. "Discussing Systemic Racism and Racial Privilege at a Large, Academic Health Center Using a Modified Privilege Walk." *BMC Med Educ* 24 (1): 327. 10.1186/s12909-024-05302-8

Carter, Genesea, and Rickie-Ann Legleitner. 2021. "Prioritizing Ourselves and Our Values: Intersectionality, Positionality, and Dismantling the Neoliberal University System." *Academic Labor: Research and Artistry* 5 (1): 1.

Chang, Brian A., Elizabeth Karin, Zachary A. Davidson, Jonathan Ripp, and Rainier P. Soriano. 2019. "Impact of a Short-Term Domestic Service-Learning Program on Medical Student Education." *Annals of Global Health* 85 (1). https://doi.org/10.5334/aogh.2465.

Chow, Candace J., Gretchen A. Case, and Cheryl E. Matias. 2019. "Tools for Discussing Identity and Privilege Among Medical Students, Trainees, and Faculty."

MedEdPORTAL: The Journal of Teaching and Learning Resources 15 (December): 10864.

"Civic Knowledge Rubric." n.d. Massachusetts Department of Higher Education. https://compact.org/sites/default/files/2022-06/CivicKnowledgeRubric.pdf.

Collins, P. H., & S. Bilge. 2020. *Getting the history of intersectionality straight? In Intersectionality.* 2nd ed.: 72–100: Polity Press.

Crenshaw, Kimberlé. 2013. "Demarginalizing the Intersection of Race and Sex: A Black Feminist Critique of Antidiscrimination Doctrine, Feminist Theory and Antiracist Politics." In *Feminist Legal Theories*, edited by Karen Maschke, 23–51. Routledge.

Davis, Denise L. F., Doquyen Tran-Taylor, Elizabeth Imbert, Jeffrey O. Wong, and Calvin L. Chou. 2021. "Start the Way You Want to Finish: An Intensive Diversity, Equity, Inclusion Orientation Curriculum in Undergraduate Medical Education." *Journal of Medical Education and Curricular Development* 8 (March): 23821205211000352.

Davidai, Shai and Tom Gilovich. 2016. "The Headwinds/Tailwinds Asymmetry: An Availability Bias in Assessments of Barriers and Blessings." *Journal of Personality and Social Psychology*, 111 (6), 835–851.

Davis, Tracy, and Laura M. Harrison. 2013. *Advancing Social Justice: Tools, Pedagogies, and Strategies to Transform Your Campus.* John Wiley & Sons.

Dean, L., and R. Thorpe. 2022. "What Structural Racism Is (or Is Not) and How to Measure It: Clarity for Public Health and Medical Researchers." *American Journal of Epidemiology* 191 (July): 1521–1526.

Dean, Lorraine T., Yuehan Zhang, Rachael R. McCleary, Rahel Dawit, Roland J. Thorpe Jr, and Darrell Gaskin. 2023. "Health Care Expenditures for Black and White US Adults Living Under Similar Conditions." *JAMA Health Forum* 4 (11): e233798.

Delgado, Richard, and Jean Stefancic. 2023. *Critical Race Theory, Fourth Edition: An Introduction.* NYU Press.

Dickman, Samuel L., Adam Gaffney, Alecia McGregor, David U. Himmelstein, Danny McCormick, David H. Bor, and Steffie Woolhandler. 2022. "Trends in Health Care Use Among Black and White Persons in the US, 1963-2019." *JAMA Network Open* 5 (6): e2217383.

Dieleman, Joseph L., Carina Chen, Sawyer W. Crosby, Angela Liu, Darrah McCracken, Ian A. Pollock, Maitreyi Sahu, et al. 2021. "US Health Care Spending by Race and Ethnicity, 2002-2016." *JAMA: The Journal of the American Medical Association* 326 (7): 649–59.

Dougherty, Geoff B., Sherita H. Golden, Alden L. Gross, Elizabeth Colantuoni, and Lorraine T. Dean. 2020. "Measuring Structural Racism and Its Association With BMI." *American Journal of Preventive Medicine* 59 (4): 530–537.

Ellison, Jonte, Chris Gunther, Mary Beth Campbell, Robin English, and Cathy Lazarus. 2021. "Critical Consciousness as a Framework for Health Equity-Focused Peer Learning." *MedEdPORTAL: The Journal of Teaching and Learning Resources* 17 (April): 11145.

Gee, Gilbert C., Anna Hing, Selina Mohammed, Derrick C. Tabor, and David R. Williams. 2019. "Racism and the Life Course: Taking Time Seriously." *American Journal of Public Health* 109 (S1): S43–S47.

Hardiman, Rita. "Conceptual Overview: Rita Hardiman and Bailey Jackson Introductory Models: Pat Griffin." *Teaching for Diversity and Social Justice* (2007): 35.

Herzog, Lindsay S., Sarah R. Wright, Jason J. Pennington, and Lisa Richardson. 2021. "The KAIROS Blanket Exercise: Engaging Indigenous Ways of Knowing to Foster Critical Consciousness in Medical Education." *Medical Teacher* 43 (12): 1437–1443.

Holdren, Sarah, Yoshiko Iwai, Nicholas R. Lenze, Amy B. Weil, and Antonia M. Randolph. 2023. "A Novel Narrative Medicine Approach to DEI Training for Medical School Faculty." *Teaching and Learning in Medicine* 35 (4): 457–66.

Holm, Amanda L., Marla Rowe Gorosh, Megan Brady, and Denise White-Perkins. 2017. "Recognizing Privilege and Bias: An Interactive Exercise to Expand Health Care Providers' Personal Awareness." *Academic Medicine: Journal of the Association of American Medical Colleges* 92 (3): 360–364.

hooks, bell. 1984. *Feminist Movement to End Violence.* South End Press.

Jindal, Monique, Rachel L. J. Thornton, Ashlyn McRae, Ndidi Unaka, Tiffani J. Johnson, and Kamila B. Mistry. 2022. "Effects of a Curriculum Addressing Racism on Pediatric Residents' Racial Biases and Empathy." *Journal of Graduate Medical Education* 14 (4). 407–413.

Johnson, A. J., ed. 2005a. "How Systems of Privilege Work." In *Privilege, Power, and Difference: 2nd Edition*, 91. McGraw-Hill.

Jones, C. P. 2000. "Levels of Racism: A Theoretic Framework and a Gardener's Tale." *American Journal of Public Health* 90 (8): 1212–1215.

Ladkin, Donna, and Joana Probert. 2021. "From Sovereign to Subject: Applying Foucault's Conceptualization of Power to Leading and Studying Power within Leadership." *Leadership Quarterly* 32 (4): 101310.

Lukachko, Alicia, Mark L. Hatzenbuehler, and Katherine M. Keyes. 2014. "Structural Racism and Myocardial Infarction in the United States." *Social Science & Medicine* 103 (February): 42–50.

Martinez, Sarah, Joseph Araj, Symone Reid, Jeslyn Rodriguez, Mytien Nguyen, Dorcas Boahema Pinto, Pamela Y. Young, Anicia Ivey, Alexis Webber, and Hyacinth Mason. 2021. "Allyship in Residency: An Introductory Module on Medical Allyship for Graduate Medical Trainees." *MedEdPORTAL: The Journal of Teaching and Learning Resources* 17 (December): 11200.

McIntosh, P. 1988. "White Privilege and Male Privilege: A Personal Account of Coming to See Correspondences through Work in Women's Studies." Working paper no. 189. Wellesley Centers for Women. http://www.nationalseedproject.org/images/documents/White_Privilege_and_Male_Privilege_Personal_Account-Peggy_McIntosh.pdf.

Merriam-Webster. n.d. "Oppression." Accessed March 9, 2024. merriam-webster.com.

Morales, Eric César. 2020. "Building Racial Coalitions: Limitations and New Directions to Teaching 'White Privilege.'" *Race and Pedagogy Journal: Teaching and Learning for Justice* 4 (3): 3.

Morgan, Kathryn Pauly. 1996. "Describing the Emperor's New Clothes: Three Myths of Educational (in)equality." In *The Gender Question in Education: Theory, Pedagogy and Politics*, edited by Ann Diller, Barbara Houston, Kathryn Pauly Morgan, and Maryann Ayim, 272. Westview. https://doi.org/10.4324/9780429496530.

Nyhan, Brendan and Jason Reifler 2010. "When Corrections Fail: The Persistence of Political Misperceptions." *Political Behavior, 32 (2)*, 303–330.

Shawar, Yusra Ribhi, and Jennifer Prah Ruger. 2019. "The Politics of Global Health Inequalities." *The Oxford Handbook of Global Health Politics* 59.

Siemers, Kyle, and Denyelle Kenyon. 2022. "Expanding SSOM's Health Equity Curriculum: Offering the Social Identities Workshop in New Student Orientation." *South Dakota Medicine: The Journal of the South Dakota State Medical Association* 75 (suppl 8): s23.

Sojourner Truth. 1851. "Ain't I a Woman." https://www.sojournertruth.com/p/aint-i-woman.html.

Wallace, Maeve, Joia Crear-Perry, Lisa Richardson, Meshawn Tarver, and Katherine Theall. 2017. "Separate and Unequal: Structural Racism and Infant Mortality in the US." *Health & Place* 45 (May): 140–144.

Williams, David R., Jourdyn A. Lawrence, and Brigette A. Davis. 2019. "Racism and Health: Evidence and Needed Research." *Annual Review of Public Health* 40: 105–25.

Witten, Nash A. K., and Gregory G. Maskarinec. 2015. "Privilege as a Social Determinant of Health in Medical Education: A Single Class Session Can Change Privilege Perspective." *Hawai'i Journal of Medicine & Public Health: A Journal of Asia Pacific Medicine & Public Health* 74 (9): 297–301.

Wu, Diana, Lamercie Saint-Hilaire, Andrew Pineda, Danielle Hessler, George W. Saba, René Salazar, and Nwando Olayiwola. 2019. "The Efficacy of an Antioppression Curriculum for Health Professionals." *Family Medicine* 51 (1): 22–30.

Zanders, Dante', and James D. Colquitt. 2023. "Use of a Discussion Provoking Board Game for Revealing Privilege." *American Journal of Surgery* 226 (4): 508–514.

Chapter 2
Power: A Foundational Look

Keilah A. Jacques

To clearly understand and act upon the multilayered and interlocked social and biological processes that determine health, public health practitioners need tools to see, name, and contextualize power structures, as well as to understand how power influences health and health inequities. Embracing the complex and multifaceted pathways through which health and the social determinants of health are influenced by the form and function of power is transformative for public health theory and practice (Schulz et al. 2020). As a newer field of study, public health has a shorter history of examining power's role in society than the fields of political and social science. For example, in the study of political movements, scholars have often defined power as the ability to influence, define, direct, and determine behavior as a result of having access to resources (Amenta, Andrews, and Caren 2018; Battilana and Casciaro 2021; Ladkin 2021). However, defining systems of power in relationship to health requires consideration of the sociopolitical agreements or relationships between individuals and institutions and the ability of agents of power to direct the definitions, resources, opportunities, and pathways to health (Shawar et al. 2019).

Examining relationships makes power visible. This chapter uses the ecological model to frame the concept of relationships and how they are formed to generate or limit power. The ecological model encompasses an examination of individuals and the systems within which they are situated while also inspecting the relationship between the two, ultimately offering a conceptual tool for organizing and evaluating population health. Ecological theories like that of Urie Bronfenbrenner are often used to guide public health research and policy (Bronfenbrenner 1978). Here, the ecological domains are defined as levels: the microsystem level, which includes an individual's interior and their immediate environment; the mesosystem[1]

---

[1] mezzosystem, is often used interchangeably in the field.

Keilah A. Jacques, *Power: A Foundational Look*. In: *Power, Privilege, and Public Health in the United States.*
Edited by: Lorraine T. Dean and Keilah A. Jacques, Oxford University Press. © Oxford University Press (2025).
DOI: 10.1093/9780197760956.003.0002

level, which includes relationships between social settings and social players such as home, school, and peer groups; and the macrosystem level, which includes interrelated relationships to societal institutions, policies, laws, rules, and norms (Bronfenbrenner 1978). When relationships are referenced, it is through this lens and with the understanding that each level is interconnected and bound to impact the other because of the interrelated nature of power dynamics.

Power is not always intrinsically harmful, problematic, or seeking manipulation. Power can take on varied forms and dimensions. Differentiating between the forms of power helps to clarify how power functions in the aforementioned relationship between actors and institutions and to clarify who is served by the form and functions in the ecological context (Haugaard 2012). Additionally, observing the conditions and influences of power in the lives and choices of people allows tracking across ecological domains (microsystem, mesosystem, and macrosystem) and contextualizes the tangible and perceived ways power is built, maximized, minimized, and maintained.

Forms of Power

Power is defined based on the relationships between actors (see Table 2.1). The most common understanding of power in the Western imagination is **power-over.** The function of power in this form is asymmetric and often coercive, requiring actors or groups to occupy a position of dominance or subordination; belonging among other relational dynamics is ordered by the dominant group (Battilana and Casciaro 2021; Ladkin 2021; Pansardi and Bindi 2021). Structurally oppressive power is here defined as a power-over. Power of this type functions relationally inside ideology-based rules and predetermined guidance that constrain and dictate the formal and informal codes in economics, political systems, educational systems, and social roles—advancing the benefits of certain groups while disadvantaging others (Cairney and Kwiatkowski 2017; Friel 2021).

Alternatively, power can be supportive and transformative in form. For example, **power-to** is an emancipatory form of power that functions to maintain the actor's ability to exert influence toward a desired outcome supporting each person in shaping their world (Harris et al. 2020; Pansardi and Bindi 2021). **Power-with** is a form of power that functions from a power-even stance. As a coactive form of power, the function is concerned with coalition building, collective strength, and advocating for collective well-being (Harris et al. 2020; Pansardi and Bindi 2021). Finally, **power-within** is a form of

Table 2.1 Forms, functions, and examples of power in the classroom

Form of power	Functional definition	Example in a classroom setting
Power-over	The function of power in this form is asymmetric and often coercive, requiring actors or groups to occupy a position of dominance or subordination; belonging among other relational dynamics is ordered by the dominant group (Pansardi and Bindi 2021; Harris et al. 2020).	• Fountain of knowledge or banking model of education, where the instructor is the main source of epistemological expertise • Exam-only assessments • Dominate voices/examples/ideals represented in the text or as examples
Power-to	Functions to maintain the actor's ability to exert influence toward a desired outcome supporting each person to shape their world (Pansardi and Bindi 2021; Harris et al. 2020).	• Competency-based learning • Dialectical learning • Un-grading formative and summative assessments
Power-with	Functions from a power-even stance; concerned with coalition-building, collective strength, and advocating for collective well-being (Pansardi and Bindi 2021; Harris et al. 2020).	• Flipped classroom approaches that allow students to actively lead discussion • Service-learning/community-based teaching • Coeducation with community representatives or colleagues who hold lived expertise
Power-within	Functions as inherent dignity and self-assuredness through self-knowledge, power of self-determination (Pansardi and Bindi 2021; Harris et al. 2020).	• Praxis models • Self-reflection activities that encourage personal connection between self and content

power that functions as inherent dignity and self-assuredness through self-knowledge, the ability of self-determination—"transformation of individual consciousness which leads to a new self-confidence to act" (Pansardi and Bindi 2021, 67) and proceeds power-with (Harris et al. 2020).

Defining, let alone actively teaching, methods for disrupting structural oppression is still an emerging pedagogical strategy in public health scholarship. Locating definitions and analytical applications of power according to the above-described framing will take some time to become a standard for practice. Conversely, social science provides several ways to scope these forms of power and their function through the work of sociopolitical theory. What follows is an examination of key theories of power that make visible the function of power-over and highlight how power could work alternatively in education. The theories and theorists that follow are mostly known for their contributions to power analysis in the field of political science. However, their work deeply informs critical pedagogy—a power-disrupting approach to teaching and learning—which can be applied to public health education.

Power Theories and Theorists

Karl Marx's Theory of Power

The Marxist theory of power is a theoretical framework that posits the existence of power structures that are deeply embedded by the ruling class into culture and nation-state politics to control the working class (Parkin 1979). According to this theory, the ruling class owns the means of production, accumulates capital, and wields power through the state to exert power over the working class (Harris et al. 2020). In essence, the ruling class uses its economic and political power to maintain the status quo and perpetuate its dominance.

The concept of hegemony comes to us from the Marxist school of thought. Hegemony is the idea that the dominant group uses cultural and social institutions to maintain their power over other groups. Hegemonic advancement is an acculturation function of power-over, which operates through consent rather than coercion or physical violence (Fonseca 2016). To this end, institutions help to shape the dominant culture, which reinforces the existing power structures and creates a sense of social order that serves the interests of the ruling class. The idea of hegemony was further developed by the Italian Marxist philosopher Antonio Gramsci, who argued that the ruling class maintains its dominance by controlling not only the economic and political spheres but also the cultural sphere (Fonseca 2016). Gramsci believed that cultural institutions could be used to create a counterhegemony, which would challenge the dominant ideology and pave the way for a more democratic and egalitarian society (Fonseca 2016).

Michel Foucault's Theory of Power

Michel Foucault's theory of power is a complex and nuanced understanding of how power is constituted through various forms of knowledge, scientific understanding, and what we consider to be "truth" in the macrosystems of our society (Gaventa 2003; Ladkin and Probert 2021). According to Foucault, there is a close relationship between power and knowledge, with power being exerted through various systems of thought and discourse—the power-over due to epistemology. These power/knowledge dynamics are reinforced through scientific discourse and institutions, outlined and profiled through the education system, the media, and political and economic ideologies—all ways of knowing and being known (Flyvbjerg 2001). Foucault's concept of disciplinary power states that society is disciplined and regulated through the threat of surveillance and visibility (Arts and Van Tatenhove 2004). This discipline is achieved without the use of outright violence but by cultural coercion and by instilling a sense of conformity and adherence to certain rules and norms. Foucault's observations of institutions illustrate how power functions in society. For this reason, disciplinary power was a key mechanism for maintaining social order and control in a power-over model.

Pierre Bourdieu's Theory of Power

Pierre Bourdieu, in *Distinction* (Bourdieu 1986) saw power as socially constructed, not simply a fixed entity or a static force. According to Bourdieu, power is created through the interplay between structure and agency and is affected by a variety of factors, including cultural norms, social class, and access to resources (Bourdieu 2023). One of the key concepts in Bourdieu's theory is the notion of "habitus," or culture. This refers to the way that socialized norms and preferences become embedded in society over time, shaping the way that individuals behave, perceive the world, and interact with others (Harris et al. 2020). Habitus is seen as a key factor in the creation and maintenance of power relations, as it influences the way that individuals perceive their position within society and how they interact with others. Another important concept in Bourdieu's theory is "cultural capital" (Harris et al. 2020). This idea refers to how access to cultural resources, such as education, art, and literature, can inform power relations within society. Those who have access to these resources, particularly those who have generational access to them, are often able to relationally use them to gain greater social and economic power, while those who lack access to these resources are often disadvantaged in terms of their social mobility and their ability to influence society (Bourdieu 2023).

Queer/Black Feminist Theories of Power

Queer/Black feminist theories of power emphasize the importance of intersectionality in comprehending the function of dominating power and offer a fresh perspective on how multiple identities intersect and are shaped by power-over structures. According to these theories proposed by influential scholars such as the members of the Combahee River Collective (Barbara and Beverly Smith, Cheryl Clarke, Demita Frazier, Audre Lorde, Marilyn James); and third wave black/ queer feminist like Chirlane McCray, Margo Okazawa-Rey, Gloria Akasha Hull, Patricia Hill Collins, Kimberlé Crenshaw, and bell hooks (Collins 2022; Combahee River Collective 1986; Crenshaw 2013; hooks 1989), power operates at various levels, and its effects are often interwoven with other social, economic, and cultural factors (Crenshaw 2013; hooks 1989).

These theories also emphasize the significance of recognizing the impact of socially ascribed power on different groups of people, particularly those who have been marginalized and oppressed by dominant power structures. They note the intersection of race, gender, and sexuality creates a unique experience of oppression that cannot be fully captured by traditional power analyses (Collins 2022; Crenshaw 2013; hooks 1989). They recognize that although power-over is about control and dominance, power-with and power-within are about resistance, agency, creativity, and solidarity (Collins 2022). These theories challenge traditional power structures or binary systems and instead focus on the experiences of marginalized individuals and communities. They also acknowledge that power is relational and contextual, and it operates differently in various spaces and contexts (Crenshaw 1989; hooks 1989). Furthermore, these theories prioritize the importance of language and discourse in shaping power dynamics, emphasizing the need for language that is inclusive and affirming of all identities and experiences. Therefore, institutions of socialization such as political, religious, and traditional education systems, which are built on and designed to perpetuate White-bodied, patriarchal, colonial, provisioned, anti-Black, antiqueer, and capitalist values to reinforce systemic oppression, needed radical interruption (Crenshaw 1989; hooks 1989). Queer/Black feminists contend that education should be more inclusive, centering the experiences and knowledge of marginalized communities and actively working against racism, sexism, and capitalism (Collins 2022; Crenshaw 1989; hooks 1989). They advocate for an education system that empowers students to challenge and transform existing power structures that perpetuate inequality and oppression. Black feminists also argue that education should cultivate critical consciousness, which is the ability to analyze and challenge existing power structures and systems of oppression by finding value in inherent worth and dignity (Crenshaw 1989; hooks 1989). By doing so, education can become a tool for liberation and justice.

Understanding Power Structures Is Critical to Health Equity Training

The interplay between power and health equity often directs attention to the distribution of health outcomes among different groups and the social determinants surrounding the health of those groups (Al-Rimawi et al. 2018; Harris et al. 2020). Health inequities refer to the "differences in health, that are not only unnecessary and avoidable but are considered unfair and unjust as they implicate power differentials in ecological relationships" (Al-Rimawi et al. 2018). Health professionals perpetuate disparities when they are unaware of, fail to respond to, or lack the skill to understand the circumstances and forces of power, even in their service provision. Without the ability to analyze the power differentials between groups, public health strategy misses key context for effective policy, practice, and research by centering individual responsibility and behavior change. A power analysis is needed to refocus interventions on root causes as opposed to the symptoms of structural inequality (Braveman 2014). Health educators have a critical role to play in addressing upstream factors, by naming and illustrating them in the classroom. If the field looks to address health inequity, educators must also provide learners with tools to consider the full range of context and root cause impacts on health like power. Critical consciousness is the ability to identify and question power's upstream role in downstream issues. Instructors who build critical consciousness prepare public health practitioners with the perspectives needed to understand, address, and consider the distribution of power at work bidirectionally for the issues of health. However, developing a multidirectional analysis is challenging if one never comes to understand the relationships or ecology of power.

For thirty years, a select number of public health scholars have worked to illuminate power by mapping different forms of oppression in health systems and the larger American society. Scholars such as Camara P. Jones and David Williams have been unflinching in calling the field to action on addressing root-cause issues (i.e., bias and racism) and defining their impacts (Jones 2002, 2019; Williams 2000, 2015). What then is the obstruction to action for public health practitioners and researchers to address issues of power? This chapter names the learning environment. As theories have pointed out, schools play a pivotal role in forging the skills of health leaders and shaping perspectives on policy, practice, and research (Schulz et al. 2020). When surveyed, instructors often agreed with the importance of examining issues of power, oppression, and differences in the social determinants of health (Karani et al. 2017; Sotto-Santiago et al 2020). However, when asked to address key issues such as this in the classroom, educators confessed that they do not have the tools or insight to carry the desire forward (Karani et al. 2017; Sotto-Santiago et al, 2020).

Prioritizing the conversation about power and privilege in the classroom may feel revolutionary and transgressive. Recent political battles over the learning environment have led to the exclusion of Black history, queer voices, and nondominant book topics or critical race theory at the K–12 levels. Though graduate curricula have not seen the same moratorium on critical consciousness development in the classroom, it has seen the defunding, dismantling, firing, and demotion of faculty who have centered on equity and historical accuracy issues. Despite the desire to squelch dissenting perspectives, critical pedagogy scholars and activists of the past championed education that contended with dominant hegemonies and provided theories and practices that are unapologetic and directive. From them, we learn how to take up the mantle of examining the role of power in the learning environment while shifting the power dynamic toward liberatory expression.

Critical Pedagogy Theorists and Power in the Learning Environment

Key thinkers in critical pedagogy, such as Carter G. Woodson, Paulo Freire, bell hooks, and Joy James, point to social-political agreements in academic institutions that are inherently shaped by power-over strategies. Critical pedagogy theorists argue that power systems work together to further dominate ideological forces at all levels of society, especially in the sociopolitical agreements of populations and the social relationships of institutions (Hall 2019). "Education either functions as an instrument which is used to facilitate the integration of the younger generation into the logic of the present system and bring about conformity, or it becomes the practice of freedom, how men and women deal critically and creatively with reality and discover how to participate in the transformation of their world" (Freire 1970). This quote highlights the ecology at play—the interconnected role of individual actors (educators) within the institutions of learning, as well as hegemonic strategies used to train learners to perpetuate the existing systems of power. To gain insight into how to alchemize power centered on domination, we examine the work of these scholars and make connections between their practice and the power analysis of previous theories. Doing so will establish a foundation for a conceptual framework that health profession educators can use to address the power gap in the teaching and learning relationship.

Louis Althusser

Louis Althusser, a prominent philosopher and Marxist theorist, has argued that dominant ideas and values in society are not natural or objective but, rather, are constructed within specific historical and social contexts. In his view, schools are a prime example of what he calls "ideological state apparatuses"—institutions that play a critical role in maintaining existing power structures and reinforcing social inequalities to further the power of and foster compliance with the state. According to Althusser, schools function primarily through the dissemination and persuasion of particular ideas and values, which serve to reinforce existing power relations and teach students to take on the role of powerless workers and maintain the status quo of dominance and subordination based on their social and political location. Althusser argues that "ideas and values are often taken for granted and accepted as natural, rather than being recognized as products of a specific historical and social context," and as such, schools operate through persuasion and coercion (Althusser 1971). In his seminal work, "Ideology and Ideological State Apparatuses," Althusser takes a power-to orientation to education and highlights the importance of understanding the role of education in shaping social consciousness in a way that aligns with dominant ideologies, to redirect them (Althusser 1971).

Carter G. Woodson

The revolutionary historian and educator Carter G. Woodson was greatly influenced by Althusser and set out to build a pedagogical affront in and outside the classroom that repurposed education as a tool for liberation and social change (Givens 2021). Though not formally recognized as a forefather of critical pedagogy, Woodson believed that education should illuminate dominant systems of power. He trained educators to empower marginalized communities through subversive pedagogies and challenge dominant narratives that perpetuate anti-Black racism and inequality (Grant, Brown, and

Brown 2015). Working from a power-within orientation, he saw White-led education boards, and state policy as "slave masters of the mind" and teachers as "fugitives" or agents of change who could work as disruptors and create alternative narratives not only with their teaching but through their lives. He built collaborations and teacher networks that trained educators to center the experiences and perspectives of marginalized communities in their instruction and advocacy (Grant, Brown, and Brown 2015). He saw the role of teachers as critical to the liberation of marginalized communities. Jarvis Givens's examination of Woodson's legacy (Woodson 2023) acknowledges that his power analysis was not limited to the classroom but extended to broader social and political contexts (e.g., a promotion of Negro history week, which is now Black History Month). He believed that teachers who were committed to collective liberation had a responsibility to engage in activism and advocacy as counteragents to the state and arbiters of a more just and equitable society (Givens, 2021).

Paulo Freire

Paulo Freire was a Brazilian philosopher, activist, and educator best known for his published work, *Pedagogy of the Oppressed*. Freire was influenced by Marx's school of thought. He coined the phrase "critical pedagogy" as a philosophical orientation to education and social movements that believed educators should encourage learners to examine power differentials in systems and patterns of oppression across social identities and economic groups (Freire 1970). Working often from a power-with stance, Freire believed education should be a means of empowering individuals and communities to challenge and overcome the oppressive structures of society and engage the learning environment as ground zero for organizing Brazilian citizens (Giroux 2005). He coined the term the "banking model" as a form of power-over: educators deposited information into the empty minds of learners, elevating the instructor to a position of all-knowing, authoritarian leader (Freire 1970). Freire argues that traditional education is based on a model of power as control, where the teacher holds all the power and the students are expected to comply (Freire 1970). The traditional model of education reinforces this false consciousness by suppressing critical thinking and encouraging conformity.

Freire alternatively believed in a power-to approach to education that was participatory and dialogical. Freire believed critical reflection and competency-based learning should work, in tandem, through praxis. In the praxis model, students are encouraged to reflect critically on their own experiences and to engage in dialogue with their peers and instructors to cocreate knowledge (Freire 1970). Through this process of dialogue and reflection, students can develop a deeper understanding of themselves and the world around them and begin to take action to address injustices. Praxis requires a shift in power dynamics (from power-over to power-with and power-within). Instructors become facilitators of learning rather than a source of knowledge (Freire 1970). Moreover, instructors work collaboratively with students to identify the issues that are important to them and to develop strategies for addressing those issues. He believed that education should be a tool for liberation and empowerment, helping individuals to recognize their agency and ability to effect change in the world (Freire 1970; Giroux 2005). He admonished instructors not to default to presenting knowledge as static. Instead, education for liberation encouraged learners to examine power differences and work toward social justice and equality (Freire and Shor 1987).

bell hooks

bell hooks, a prominent feminist scholar and social activist, developed a comprehensive philosophy on power and education because she engaged with Freire's work. Like Freire, she emphasized the importance of utilizing education as a tool to challenge and transform systems of oppression, especially "imperial, patriarchal, colonial, white supremacist, racist, misogynistic" forms of oppression (hooks 2014). She dialogues with Freire about the gap in his approach by naming the role of patriarchy and sexism in his analysis of power. Therefore, she advocated for a pedagogy of liberation that encourages critical thinking, dialogue, and a recognition of the interconnectedness of all forms of oppression. hooks saw love as an essential ingredient in education. She believed it allows students to bring their full humanity to the learning environment and contextualize the intersectional self (both instructor and learner) in the learning environment. Her work asserts that doing so helps learners and instructors feel welcomed and supported, enabling them to engage with learning in a meaningful way (hooks 1994). hooks's work in education often focuses on power-within. Her definition of love is grounded in inherent human dignity, which she believed enabled instructors and learners to build connections with others across differences and identify similarities (hooks 1989). To this end, self-reflection served as another key component of hooks's power analysis in education. She emphasizes the importance of self-awareness and critical reflection in the learning process, arguing that students must learn to examine their own biases, beliefs, and assumptions to develop a deeper understanding of themselves and the world around them (hooks 2014). By engaging in self-reflection, students can challenge their own biases and prejudices and develop a more nuanced and empathetic understanding of others. This approach to education promotes active engagement with, rather than passive acceptance of, power differentials. It seeks to empower individuals to become agents of change in their own lives and society as a whole.

Joy James

Joy James is a respected researcher, theologian, and philosopher who writes extensively on the interplay between power and education. In her works on academia, James argues that academia serves as an "anti-revolutionary formation" that reinforces existing power structures (James 2003). According to James, academic institutions are designed to uphold and maintain the dominant ideologies of society (James 2003). This means that academia often fails to challenge the dominant narratives and can even actively discourage dissenting voices. James's work points out the role of academic institutions in promoting conformity and discouraging critical thinking (Grewal 1994; James 2003). She argues that the academic publishing industry, for example, reinforces the status quo by prioritizing research that aligns with existing theories and perspectives. This can lead to a lack of diversity in academic discourse and a failure to address important social issues. To counter the power-over function of education, James advocates for a more inclusive and democratic approach to research that promotes critical thinking and encourages students to question dominant narratives. James emphasizes key intellectual activities that combine theory and practice, to not only critique existing power structures but also to actively work to dismantle them through grassroots organizing and political activism, which may result in violence between the activist and the academic institution and, further, the state (James 2003, 2010). She argues that this power-to approach can help students develop a more nuanced understanding of power dynamics and their role in perpetuating or challenging them. James also emphasizes the importance of recognizing the radical intersectionality of power and the role of maternal contributors to social change. She accomplishes this by challenging academics to consider the role of violence inside the institution and within the state (James 1998; Grewal 1994). According to James, activist intellectuals are individuals who not only engage in intellectual work but also use their knowledge and expertise to bring about social, political, and economic change (Grewal 1994; James 1998, 2003, 2010).

Education as a Tool for Domination and Disruptive Opportunities for the Instructor

All of these scholars share the belief that education is often used as a tool to perpetuate dominant power structures where one group has power over another. They argue that this binary power structure is based on dominance and subordination. However, they also believe that the learning environment can be transformed and lead to liberation when instructors subvert dominant ideals, culture, and codes through critical pedagogy. Additionally, each scholar makes a statement on the role of instructors and highlights the ways power takes on a form and functions across various ecological levels simultaneously. For example, examining the microlevel of power involves inspecting the *inter*personal and *intra*personal interactions of educators. Here, power in a dominant form centers the ego by operating from the banking model of education. This model views the learner as an object who receives the educator's agenda for learning, requiring that the status quo remains.

These critical scholars provide guidance and pragmatic approaches to move the pedagogy and practice of power analysis forward in the learning environment, as summarized in Figure 2.1. From their work and lives comes

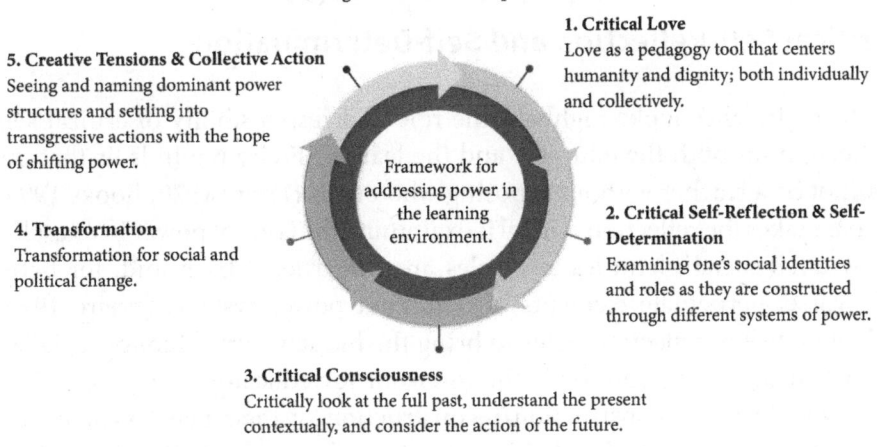

Teaching & Power: A Conceptual Model

5. Creative Tensions & Collective Action
Seeing and naming dominant power structures and settling into transgressive actions with the hope of shifting power.

4. Transformation
Transformation for social and political change.

Framework for addressing power in the learning environment.

1. Critical Love
Love as a pedagogy tool that centers humanity and dignity; both individually and collectively.

2. Critical Self-Reflection & Self-Determination
Examining one's social identities and roles as they are constructed through different systems of power.

3. Critical Consciousness
Critically look at the full past, understand the present contextually, and consider the action of the future.

Figure 2.1 Teaching & power: a conceptual model.
Source: Conceptualized and designed by the author.

the following conceptual framework for addressing power in teaching and learning that develops liberatory education and supports skill development for health equity.

Critical Love

Love as a pedagogy tool is given to us formally by bell hooks but comes from her understanding of the often cited civil rights motivation articulated best in Dr. Martin Luther King Jr's 1967 speech "Where Do We Go From Here," where King asserts, "Power without love is reckless and abusive, and love without power is sentimental and anemic. Power at its best is love implementing the demands of justice, and justice at its best is power correcting everything that stands against love" (King 2010).

Neither King nor hooks is speaking of love in the romantic sense but of love that is deeply rooted in care for humanity, human dignity, and motivation. The foundation of any pedagogy that is committed to addressing systems of power must be grounded in love for humanity and care for the human experience in such a way that it will see injustice and act to further justice. Furthermore, it promotes humility that reminds the instructor that they are not the center of the learning universe and invites them to collaborate with students in curating a learning opportunity that benefits everyone involved. When modeled, that commitment to humanity becomes the standard of practice for students as they leave the learning environment and enter the world.

Critical Self-Reflection and Self-Determination

Both Freire and hooks highlight the role and responsibility of critical self-reflection for both the educator and the learner. Freire reminds us that one cannot be a teacher without exposing who one is (Freire 1970; hooks 1994). What makes the reflection critical is examining the issue of power in oneself—how one's social identities and roles are constructed by it and, for better or worse, perpetuate elements of dominant power systems (Freire 1970). The practice of reflection helps to bring the hidden curriculum of socialization and dominant culture to the forefront for educators and forces them to invest in the deconstruction/reconstruction of their belief systems and subsequent actions in the classroom, before, during, and after they engage learners (Giroux 1983, 2005). It also encourages them to create spaces for critical self-reflection in the learning environment—prompts learners to think about their origin stories, socialization, and power-related identities and incorporate analysis of self into analysis of other systems.

Critical self-reflection works in tandem with self-determination. Analyzing systems of power can promote self-determination by providing a learning environment that inspires learners to shape their own learning sphere, express dissenting thoughts, and create cultures grounded in their experiences. Ultimately, classrooms must become brave spaces where learners can resist oppression safely, confidently, and frequently. As hooks (1994) notes, self-determination enables us to resist oppressive forces. Joy James (2010) argues that self-determination is not just about individual autonomy but is also about collective agency and the ability of marginalized communities to define their own goals and strategies for liberation. Learners need to be able to analyze their experiences and the world around them critically to take action and transform their reality. Freire (1970) suggests that the more individuals become aware of their oppression and its nature, the more they are convinced of their task to free themselves. Self-determination builds on other elements of the framework and is enhanced by critical consciousness-raising activities and identifying opportunities for resistance and transformation. Critical pedagogy is foundational in supporting learners in understanding the power that works against their survival and the power their communities have to engage in change. Self-determination highlights the importance of power-within and power-to. Individual agency begets collective agency, which challenges systems of oppression and achieves power shifts. However, the ability to identify one's own goals and values is essential in laying the foundation for interest convergence, collective strategies for liberation, and alliances across groups.

Critical Consciousness (Historical Analysis)

Carter G. Woodson led the way on critical consciousness development in word and action. Again, the critical component is the invitation to examine power dynamics, but for Woodson, this was overlaid with a historical analysis. In his 1933 work *The Mis-Education of the Negro*", he is noted for stating, "Those who have no record of what their forebears have accomplished lose the inspiration which comes from the teaching of biography and history" (Woodson, 2023). For him, teaching required the ability to look at the past fully, understand the present contextually, and consider the action of the future from this informed state. Freire and hooks highlight the responsibility of the instructor in curating culturally and historically accurate depictions of history in the power analysis. It is Joy James, however, who reminds us that educators committed to widening the historical lens and canon to be inclusive of nondominant stories, or instructors who ask learners to critically analyze the role of power, are not guaranteed safety in the future. Academia is hostile to those who take up this practice. And yet, this risky responsibility is both necessary and revolutionary. Critical consciousness gave us thinkers like Dr. Martin Luther King Jr. and Malcolm X—whose ethic of love led them to conflict with the state, in the name of justice. It gave us The Black Panthers and the Young Lords, whose revolutionary action produced the Patient Bill of Rights and federally qualified health centers as access points in health. But it also cost those revolutionaries their lives and livelihoods. Freire was banned from his country of origin, and hooks was ostracized from many academic communities.

Transformation

The activation of critical love, critical self-reflection, and critical conscious-ness brings about a fundamental shift that enables an individual to perceive the world more completely and take necessary actions to transform it. This transformation, as a present activity is essential for social and political change and is a process of liberation from oppression and domination (James 2003). Dialogue in the learning environment and critical reflection support transfor-mation, but Freire emphasized that true education is only rhetoric if it lacks real-world application. Educators have a responsibility to facilitate the intense development process and provide learners with praxis and real-world appli-cations. Praxis is the cycle of learning, doing, acting, and reflecting to create meaning, then repeated into perpetuity. Transformation requires a willing-ness to challenge existing power structures and work toward power-with that functions to create a more equitable and just society.

Creative Tension and Collective Action

Education is the process of conscientization where marginalized individuals become aware of their oppression. Creative tension, a concept borrowed from the Dr. Martin Luther King, Jr.'s "Letter from Birmingham Jail" (King 1964), is about being in a relationship with the discomfort that results from seeing and naming dominant power structures and settling into transgressive actions, with the hope of igniting ideological shifts. Instructors can both model and support creative tension in the learning environment through the practice of interrogation and problem-solving; not just with and for those at the margins but in solidarity and collective struggle for liberation. Freire and hooks highlight the role of collective problem-solving through questions and discussion that draw connections to collective futures (Freire 2000; hooks 2014). Co-creation of knowledge through the practices of dialectics and praxis engages in interrogating power and innovation solutions (power-with) that develop solidarity across groups. Freire (2000), in particular, speaks to the role of group reflection in developing a shared consciousness of their sociopolitical location and strategy development for change. Carter G. Woodson believed that collective action was essential for achieving social and political change in America. He argued that individuals could not achieve equality on their own, but needed to work together to challenge the structures of oppression that existed in American society (Woodson 1933). Similarly, Joy James (2013) argues that collective action is a process by which individuals come together to address a common issue or challenge. Here, learning is completed in the action, advanced to collective results.

What is the field of public health, if not the call to creative tension and collective action to shift the power dynamics and increase quality of life and life expectancy? By working together, individuals can leverage shared resources, skills, and knowledge to achieve a common goal of health. Similarly, teaching students to both recognize and understand oppressive systems, educators must prime them to seek out solutions that build solidarity, share resources, and amplify the voices of the most marginalized—past, present, and future. Dr. King's collective tension invites us to see collective action as a standard for practice in teaching and learning. Instructors can help students look at histories of collective action and their impact on current power relationships.

Teaching the next generation of public health leaders about past ways marginalized groups challenged dominant narratives, demanded accountability from those in power, and transformed oppressive health systems is to teach a complete history of health movements.

Taken together, the elements within the conceptual frameworks serve as a guide for instructors to see, name, and contextualize the form and functions of power broadly, as well as to examine the role of power in teaching and learning. Each element illustrates power across form and function, ecological systems, and levels of consideration for a personal and professional orientation to how power is used, shifts, challenges, and changes. Moreover, it guides instructors, practitioners, and researchers to reflect on how power influences their pedagogy practices and serves as scaffolding for analyzing the sociopolitical systems and structures that form the context for illness and health. This chapter invites readers to lean into reflection as a step in praxis: take time to consider how you have been socialized to understand power, what definitions of power you default to in teaching and learning, and how you use power in the classroom. Additionally, the chapter works to make systems of power visible in order to shift public health professional pedagogy (philosophy and practice of teaching and learning) and curricular design (content development and implementation). The final invitation is to apply this chapter and commit to reapplying it as a liberatory practice and form of resistance to dominant power in teaching and learning.

References

Al-Rimawi, R., J. Alshraideh, and M. Al-Hussami. 2018. "Historical Development of Health Equity: Literature Review." *International Journal of Applied and Natural Sciences (IJANS)* 7 (1): 27–34.

Althusser, L. 1971. "Ideology and Ideological State Apparatuses (Notes Towards an Investigation)." In *Lenin and Philosophy and Other Essays*, edited by L. Althusser, 127–186. Monthly Review Press.

Amenta, E., K. T. Andrews, and N. Caren 2018. "The Political Institutions, Processes, and Outcomes Movements Seek to Influence." In *The Wiley Blackwell Companion to Social Movements*, edited by D. A. Snow, S. A. Soule, H. Kriesi, and H. J. McCammon, 237–252.

Arts, Bas, and Jan Van Tatenhove. 2004. "Policy and Power: A Conceptual Framework between the 'Old' and 'New' Policy Idioms." *Policy Sciences* 37: 339–356.

Battilana, Julie, and Tiziana Casciaro. 2021. *Power, for All: How It Really Works and Why It's Everyone's Business*. Simon and Schuster.

Bourdieu, Pierre. 1986. "The Forms of Capital." In *Handbook of Theory and Research for the Sociology of Education*, edited by J. G. Richardson, 241–258. Greenwood.

Braveman, Paula. 2014. "What Are Health Disparities and Health Equity? We Need to be Clear." *Public Health Reports* 129 (1, Suppl. 2): 5–9.

Bronfenbrenner, Urie. 1978. "Who Needs Parent Education?" *Teachers College Record* 79 (4): 1–14.

Cairney, Paul, and Richard Kwiatkowski. 2017. "How to Communicate Effectively with Policymakers: Combine Insights from Psychology and Policy Studies." *Palgrave Communications* 3 (1): 1–8.

Collins, Patricia Hill. 2022. *Black Feminist Thought: Knowledge, Consciousness, and the Politics of Empowerment*. Routledge.

Combahee River Collective. 1986. "The Combahee River Collective Statement: Black Feminist Organizing in the Seventies and Eighties." http://books.google.com/books?id=sEqaAAAAIAAJ

Crenshaw, Kimberlé. 1989. "Demarginalizing the Intersection of Race and Sex: A Black Feminist Critique of Antidiscrimination Doctrine, Feminist Theory, and Antiracist Politics." *University of Chicago Legal Forum* 1989 (1): 139–167.

Crenshaw, Kimberlé Williams. 2013. "Mapping the Margins: Intersectionality, Identity Politics, and Violence Against Women of Color." In *The Public Nature of Private Violence*, edited by Martha Albertson Fineman and Roxanne Mykitiuk, 93–118. Routledge.

Flyvbjerg, Bent. 2001. *Making Social Science Matter: Why Social Inquiry Fails and How It Can Succeed Again.* Cambridge University Press.

Fonseca, Marcio. 2016. *Gramsci's Critique of Civil Society: Towards a New Concept of Hegemony.* Routledge.

Friel, Sharon, Belinda Townsend, Max Fisher, P. Harris, T. Freeman, and F. Baum. 2021. "Power and the People's Health." *Social Science & Medicine* 282: 114173.

Freire, Paulo. 1970. *Pedagogy of the Oppressed.* Herder and Herder.

Freire, Paulo, and Ira Shor. 1987. *A Pedagogy for Liberation: Dialogues on Transforming Education.* Macmillon.

Gaventa, John. 2003. *Power after Lukes: An Overview of Theories of Power Since Lukes and Their Application to Development* 8(11): 1–18. Brighton: Participation Group, Institute of Development Studies.

Giroux, Henry A. 1983. *Theory and Resistance in Education: A Pedagogy for the Opposition.* Bergin & Garvey.

Giroux, Henry A. 2005. "Paulo Freire, Politics, and Pedagogy: Revisiting Pedagogy of the Oppressed." *Educational Researcher* 34 (3): 3–12.

Givens, J. R. 2021. *Fugitive Pedagogy: Carter G. Woodson and the Art of Black Teaching.* Harvard University Press.

Grant, C. A., K. D. Brown, and A. L. Brown. 2015. *Black Intellectual Thought in Education: The Missing Traditions of Anna Julia Cooper, Carter G. Woodson, and Alain Leroy Locke.* Routledge.

Grewal, Inderpal. 1994. "The Womb of Western Theory: Trauma, Time Theft, and the Captive Maternal." In *Theorizing Feminism: Parallel Trends in the Humanities and Social Sciences*, edited by Anne C. Herrmann and Abigail J. Stewart, 269–284. Westview Press.

Harris, Patrick, Fran Baum, Sharon Friel, T. Mackean, A. Schram, and B. Townsend. 2020. "A Glossary of Theories for Understanding Power and Policy for Health Equity." *Journal of Epidemiology and Community Health* 74 (6): 548–552.

Haugaard, Mark. 2012. "Rethinking the Four Dimensions of Power: Domination and Empowerment." *Journal of Political Power* 5 (1): 33–54.

hooks, bell. 1989. "Feminism and Black Women's Studies." *Sage* 6 (1): 54.

hooks, bell. 1994. *Teaching to Transgress: Education as the Practice of Freedom.* Routledge.

hooks, bell. 2014. *Writing Beyond Race: Living Theory and Practice*. Routledge.

James, Joy. 1998. "Theorizing Resistance to Oppression." In *Theorizing Feminisms: A Reader*, edited by Elizabeth Hackett and Sally Haslanger, 367–390. Oxford University Press.

James, Joy. 2003. "Academia, Activism, and Imprisoned Intellectuals." *Social Justice* 30 (2): 3–7.

James, Joy. 2010. *Seeking the Bellicose, the Coy, and the Outlandish: Critical Education, Black Feminist Theory, and Practice*. Routledge.

James, Joy. 2013. "Theorizing Resistance in the Age of Austerity: Radical Possibilities and Neoliberal Constraints." In *Critical Theories, IR and "The Anti-Globalisation Movement": The Politics of Global Resistance*, edited by Jenny Edkins and Bulent Diken, 44–63. Routledge.

Jones, Camara. 2002. "The Impact of Racism on Health." *Ethnicity & Disease* 12 (1): 10–13.

Jones, Camara Phyllis. 2019. *Action and Allegories*. https://doi.org/10.2105/9780875533049ch11

Karani, Reena, Lara Varpio, Win May, Tanya Horsley, John Chenault, Karen Hughes Miller, and Bridget O'Brien. 2017. "Commentary: Racism and Bias in Health Professions Education: How Educators, Faculty Developers, and Researchers Can Make a Difference." *Academic Medicine* 92 (11S): S1–S6.

King, Martin Luther Jr. 2003. "Letter from a Birmingham Jail." In *Liberating Faith: Religious Voices for Justice, Peace, & Ecological Wisdom*, edited by Roger S. Gottlieb, 177–187. Rowman & Littlefield.

King, Martin Luther Jr. 2010. *Where Do We Go from Here: Chaos or Community?* Vol. 2. Beacon Press.

Ladkin, Donna. 2021. "Problematizing Authentic Leadership: How the Experience of Minoritized People Highlights the Impossibility of Leading from One's 'True Self.'" *Leadership* 17 (4): 395–400.

Ladkin, Donna, and Joanne Probert. 2021. "From Sovereign to Subject: Applying Foucault's Conceptualization of Power to Leading and Studying Power within Leadership." *Leadership Quarterly* 32 (4): 101310.

Pansardi, Pamela, and Marianna Bindi. 2021. "The New Concepts of Power? Power-Over, Power-To and Power-With." In *Essays on Evolutions in the Study of Political Power*, edited by Giulio M. Gallarotti, 51–71. Routledge.

Parkin, Frank. 1979. *Marx's Theory of History: A Bourgeois Critique*. New York: Columbia University Press.

Schulz, Amy J., Roshanak Mehdipanah, Linda M. Chatters, A. G. Reyes, E. W. Neblett Jr, and B. A. Israel. 2020. "Moving Health Education and Behavior Upstream: Lessons from COVID-19 for Addressing Structural Drivers of Health Inequities." *Health Education & Behavior* 47 (4): 519–524.

Shawar, Yusra Ribhi, and Jennifer Prah Ruger. 2019. "The Politics of Global Health Inequalities." In *The Oxford Handbook of Global Health Politics*, edited by Colin McInnes, Kelley Lee, and Jeremy Youde, 59. Oxford University Press.

Sotto-Santiago, Sylk, Jacqueline Mac, Francesca Duncan, and Joseph Smith. 2020. "'I Didn't Know What to Say': Responding to Racism, Discrimination, and Microaggressions with the OWTFD Approach." *MedEdPORTAL* 16: 10971.

Williams, D. R., and R. Wyatt 2015. "Racial Bias in Health Care and Health: Challenges and Opportunities." *Jama* 314 (6): 555–556.

Williams, David R., and Toni D. Rucker. 2000. "Understanding and Addressing Racial Disparities in Health Care." *Health Care Financing Review* 21 (4): 75.

Woodson, C. G. 2023. *The Mis-education of the Negro*. Penguin.

Chapter 3
Examining the Coin of Privilege in Health and Healthcare

Angie Phenix, Meredith Smith, Lindsay Beavers, and Stephanie Nixon

Introduction to Antioppression and the Coin Model

In discussions of equity, diversity, and inclusion (EDI) in healthcare, we often frame the problem to be addressed as marginalized individuals or communities. However, this conceptualization fails to recognize the historic and intersecting systems of inequality that produce this marginalization. Furthermore, we typically fail to recognize that the same systems that bring harm to the health of some also actively benefit the health of others. How can we do better? One way of understanding how power operates in society is an approach known as "antioppression." Antioppression acknowledges that oppression exists and focuses on challenging the systems of oppression that create inequities (aqil et al. 2021; Lavallée 2014; Lyons et al. 2023). This approach understands all systems of oppression as interconnected and mutually reinforcing. Put another way, antioppression incorporates intersectionality, an analysis advanced by Kimberlé Crenshaw and others, which recognizes the complex arrangements of disadvantage that are produced when multiple forms of oppression intersect (Atewologun 2018; Crenshaw 2002; Lavallée 2014). Antioppression is a broad term that may encompass discussions of racism (and other "isms"), colonization, privilege, and power (Galloway et al. 2019; Harlow and Hearn 1996; Zinga and Styres 2019).

Antioppressive action commonly involves unlearning one's previous (mis-)understanding of how power operates in society and relearning a more coherent intersectional analysis. A critical and self-reflexive lens is a crucial component of antioppressive practice in order to identify one's own relationship to upholding systems of oppression—especially when one is in a position of privilege (Kumashiro 2000; Lavallée 2014).

Angie Phenix et al., *Examining the Coin of Privilege in Health and Healthcare*. In: *Power, Privilege, and Public Health in the United States*. Edited by: Lorraine T. Dean and Keilah A. Jacques, Oxford University Press. © Oxford University Press (2025). DOI: 10.1093/9780197760956.003.0003

Our experience has been that while antioppression has a long tradition in social change movements, this approach is less common within the health sphere—including within health research, practice, and policy and health profession education. The "coin model of privilege and critical allyship" was created as an effort to translate core concepts in antioppression for a health audience (Nixon 2019; Nixon 2020, 2021). In particular, the model seeks to clarify the concept of *privilege* and what to do with it in the pursuit of a more just and healthy world for all. The model was adapted from the schematic of privilege, domination, and oppression presented by Kathryn Pauly Morgan (1996).

The coin model helps bring to light how people in positions of power and privilege frequently address EDI and the needs of marginalized groups in ways that reproduce instead of uproot inequities. Our assumption here is that people drawn to healthcare are well intentioned, so this argument is unlinked from ill will. In many cases, as highlighted in Dr. Dean's chapter (Chapter 11) of this book, people's actions may be done with a desire for scientific advancement and the greater good of us all. Rather, we assert that the absence of a coherent intersectional power analysis, such as antioppression, leads many of us working in healthcare to act in ways that re-entrench as opposed to redress inequalities.

The aim of this chapter is twofold. First, we introduce the coin model as the basis for building a more coherent power analysis. Second, we use the ideas in the coin model to illustrate how actions we take in the health sphere can help move us all toward transformation as opposed to re-entrenching the status quo.

The Coin, the Top of the Coin, and the Bottom of the Coin

The coin metaphor has three parts: the coin itself, the top of the coin, and the bottom of the coin. The coin itself, depicted in Figure 3.1, represents a historic system of inequality. These are the social structures created before any of us were born that were designed by some to deploy power over others. These systems are social, meaning that they are embedded throughout society. As such, we are unable to opt out of them; we have grown up within them. They are the air we breathe.

We are talking here about the "isms," such as colonialism, racism, sexism, heterosexism, cisgenderism, ableism, and the list goes on. For example, the US and Canada are settler colonies, meaning that these nations were created through the process of colonizing Indigenous lands. There is no part

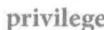

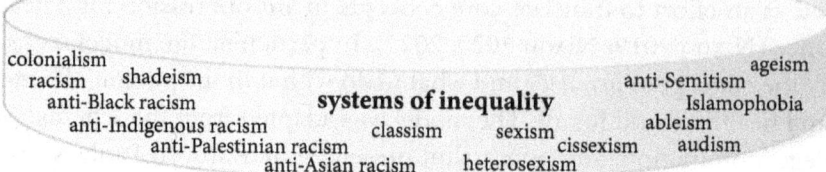

privilege
unearned advantage
you have it **because** of who you happen to be

colonialism
racism   shadeism   anti-Semitism ageism
anti-Black racism   **systems of inequality**   Islamophobia
anti-Indigenous racism   classism   sexism   ableism
anti-Palestinian racism   cissexism   audism
anti-Asian racism   heterosexism

oppression
unearned disadvantage
you have it because of who you happen to be

Figure 3.1 Coin model of privilege and critical allyship.
Source: Conceptualized and designed by the authors.

of present-day activity in Canada or the US that occurs outside that context; it is the history we have collectively inherited, and its impacts continue today, including through inequities in health that are part of the design of colonization.

Each of us finds ourselves on the top of some coins and the bottom of other coins at the same time—not because of our behavior or effort, but because of how we happen to be structured in history.

We find ourselves on the top of a coin when our social identity aligns with the historic plane of domination. We did not ask to find ourselves on the top of the coin; we just are because of who we happen to be. For instance, picking up on the example above, people who are settlers find themselves on the top of settler colonialism. People who are heterosexual (or "straight") find themselves on the top of the coin of heterosexism. People who are men find themselves on the top of the coin of sexism. People who are cisgender find themselves on the top of the coin of cissexism. People who are White find themselves on the top of the coin of racism. And people who are not Black find themselves on the top of the coin of anti-Black racism. When we find ourselves on the top of a coin, we receive benefits that others do not. We did not earn them. We may not even know we are receiving them—but we get them all the same (McIntosh 1988).

We find ourselves on the bottom of the coin when our social identity is aligned with the subordination side of the historic system of inequality. For instance, Indigenous Peoples find themselves on the bottom of the coin of settler colonialism. People who are not heterosexual find themselves on the bottom of the coin of heterosexism. People who are not men find themselves on the bottom of the coin of sexism. People who are transgender find themselves on the bottom of the coin of cissexism. People who are marginalized due to race find themselves on the bottom of the coin of racism. And people who are Black find themselves on the bottom of the coin of anti-Black racism. Importantly, the position on the bottom of the coin is not a position of weakness or victimhood. On the contrary, historic and contemporary movements for social change have been and continue to be led by communities on the bottom of coins.

Recalling intersectionality, it is crucial that we pay attention to the multiple social locations we hold at the same time, on the top of some coins and the bottom of others, in order to tune into the complex arrangements of advantage or disadvantage that will play out differently according to context. This is true for ourselves and for how we understand the experiences of our colleagues, patients, and students.

The Misdiagnosis Resulting from the Absence of a Coherent Power Analysis and How this Leads to Ineffective and Harmful Actions

Now that we have a sense of the coin, we offer a thought exercise to illustrate how quickly we can lose sight of the three components to this metaphor, leading to a misdiagnosis of the problem that needs to be addressed.

For this thought exercise, we invite readers to focus their mind's eye on the bottom of the coin—that is, the position of oppression (or unearned disadvantage) received not because of behavior but because of how one is structured in history. We then invite reflection on the general terms we have in public health (and beyond) to describe groups of people *whose outcomes are worse* because they find themselves positioned on the bottom of the coin. These general terms may include marginalized groups, disadvantaged populations, at-risk groups, vulnerable people, and the hard to reach or hard to serve.

We then invite readers to focus their mind's eye on the top of the coin—that is, the position of privilege (or unearned advantage) received not because of merit or worth but because of how one is structured in history. Again, we invite readers to name the general terms we have in public health (and beyond) to describe groups of people *whose outcomes are better* because of the unearned advantage they receive by virtue of finding themselves positioned on the top of the coin. We swiftly realize that there is not a parallel language for the top of the coin. The closest we might come to accurately naming this position is lucky populations or unfairly advantaged groups—terms that are not part of the public health lexicon. In fact, this position on the top of the coin commonly slips from being understood as unearned advantage to the inaccurate reframing of "normal," or the default, which is beyond even naming. The absence of vocabulary related to the top of the coin means we do not have a mind map for considering this part of the power analysis. By erroneously understanding these groups as "normal," we often consider people on the top of coins to be the referent groups in our quantitative analyses; we compare the health of other groups to this "norm" or "standard" without acknowledging that this is actually a position of unearned advantage.

Furthermore, our experience has been that efforts to advance justice and EDI in the health sphere not only "invisibilize" the top of the coin, but they also invisibilize the coin itself. As such, the totality of the problem that needs to be addressed through EDI becomes framed as the bottom of the coin. This is a dangerous misdiagnosis. To be clear, people on the bottom of the coin are not a problem to be fixed. The problem is the coin (i.e., the system of oppression woven into the fabric of our institutions) and the (often unwitting) complicity of people on the top of the coin in upholding these unjust systems, despite their intention to do the opposite.

How does this happen? This occurs in part because we have received lessons throughout our lives that our various positions on the top of coins are not simply social locations just like any other but, instead, are the right way to be or the default against which all others are judged to be different. We have been taught that there is no top of the coin and, therefore, that we hold a position of neutrality in relation to social justice—that is, what's happening to those marginalized communities is unjust, but it has nothing to do with me personally. However, for the coins where we find ourselves on top, we are not *neutral*; we are part and parcel of the system of oppression. There is no opting out of these coins and there is no neutral. For the coins where we are on top, we are upholding these systems of oppression until we are not.

So what might be the alternative? What might be a different orientation for action on justice and EDI within the health sphere for the coins where we find ourselves structured in history in a position of privilege?

The Reorientation for Action when We Get the Diagnosis Right

The original coin model article frames this orientation as "practicing critical allyship." Others have described this practice as being an accomplice, coconspirator, or coliberator. Regardless of naming, the spirit calls for rejecting the premise of people on the top of the coin helping or saving people on the bottom (because people on the bottom of the coin are not the problem). Rather, the shift is toward the shared aim of *collective liberation* by working across the coin to address the real problem, which is the coin—that is, the intersecting systems of oppression that are bad for all of us. The Anti-Oppression Network describes this orientation as "an active, consistent, and arduous practice of unlearning and re-evaluating, in which a person in a position of privilege and power seeks to operate in solidarity with a marginalized group" (https://theantioppressionnetwork.com/allyship/).

What might this unlearning and reevaluating involve? Our experience as clinicians, health educators, and scholars seeking to practice antioppression in our day-to-day work in healthcare has been that this is ongoing, nonlinear, iterative, and messy work in which we are constantly trying to move from the default stance we have learned and toward actions and approaches aligned with collective liberation.

This approach is in direct contrast to the message we have been taught over and over again that we are the experts in healthcare and that our role is to "fix problems." On the contrary, for coins where we find ourselves on top (i.e., in a position of privilege), we are by definition nonexperts, and part of our work is to unlearn the internalized sense of superiority that comes with this position in order to make room for the unlearning required for our authentic participation in collective action for enduring change.

How can we better understand nuances of the default stance that trick us into deploying well-intentioned actions that end up reentrenching the status quo? And what might actions look like that are aligned with a coherent power analysis and the aim of collective liberation? See Table 3.1.

Parting Thoughts

Systems of oppression, or coins, such as racism, colonialism, ableism, cissexism, and others, cause health disparities for people who experience unearned

Table 3.1 Contrasting actions in healthcare that lead toward transformation as opposed to entrenching the status quo[a]

	Entrenching the status quo	Toward transformation
The experts are:	Formal leaders in healthcare and other sectors—that is, people who hold control of the budget and policy-making, decisions • For example, settler healthcare workers are positioned as the experts in providing care to Indigenous peoples, resulting in a Western-only approach to health • For example, healthcare funding is contingent on metrics that are tied to Western-centric outcome measures	Marginalized people and communities in terms of day-to-day experiences of oppression and leaders within those communities with specific insight on dismantling unjust systems. • For example, autonomous Indigenous-led health centers that focus on providing places of health and healing guided by Indigenous versus Western worldviews
The role of people in positions of privilege is:	Neutral and disconnected from systems of inequality This means those in privilege can walk away from issues • For example, Western notions of professionalism centered on politeness and disconnectedness • Healthcare workers positioned as neutral; our life experiences are deemed irrelevant to our professional practice, and this approach is worked into healthcare training (e.g., see Lavallee & Harding 2022) • The logic is that people in positions of privilege should lead the work	Complicit and bound up in the systems of inequality • For example, people recognizing and naming their positions of privilege and actively working to leverage their unearned advantage, power, and safety to shift power to people with expertise and experience on the bottom of the coin • The logic is that people in positions of privilege should not lead the work (alone); they should recognize the expertise of those who experience the disadvantage and orient themselves in solidarity

| **The orientation and motivation for people in positions of privilege is:** | Helping, fixing, and saving marginalized people based on altruism and generosity
• People on the bottom of the coin are the problem to be addressed
• For example, healthcare workers' insistence on the normative goal of "fixing" a person so they can walk versus the patient's desire to use a wheelchair for mobility; leads to a rehabilitation plan focused on normalization and disconnected from patients' goal to participate in the world on their terms | Collective liberation
Privileged folks recognize that systems of oppression are bad for us all and work in solidarity across the coin to collectively build a future that is better for all
• The problems to be addressed are the coin and the unwitting complicity of those on top
• For example, shifting from a mentality of fixing/saving people to responding to calls to action from individuals and communities
• For example, asking what meaningful health looks like as a starting point for a treatment plan and following through with goals that align with the patient's wishes |
| **The target for action is:** | Blaming individual "bad apples"—that is, other people who are intentionally doing bad things
• The logic is to search for *if* this is happening in healthcare
• For example, microaggression workshops that are focused on stopping other people (bad apples) from doing bad things but that are not nested in a coherent power analysis of how coins are structural and embedded in healthcare and higher education. | Systems of oppression that play out in multiple ways and levels throughout the health sphere, as they were designed to do
• The logic is to start with the assumption that this *is* happening in healthcare and focus on uprooting the current and future ways it shows up
• For example, interventions at the personal/internal, interpersonal, and systemic/institutional levels |

continued

Table 3.1 *continued*

	Entrenching the status quo	Toward transformation
Accountability is:	To the institution	To the communities historically excluded and harmed by the systems of oppression
	• Leads to people in positions of privilege and without expertise related to dismantling systems of oppression being positioned as the experts to design, deliver, and fund their own solutions	• Leads to people in positions of privilege and without expertise related to dismantling systems of oppression realizing their role is to leverage their power and safety to work in solidarity with struggle leaders inside and outside the institution
		• May mean people in positions of privilege setting up additional accountability structures beyond the academy/healthcare institution to ensure they are moving accountably in relation to affected communities
The role of body, emotions, and spirit is:	Nonexistent	Fundamental
	Embodiment has no place in this approach; it is only intellectual/about the mind	Connection to body, emotion, and spirit is a prerequisite for change-making work
	• For example, the embodied and emotional resistance (in the form of guilt, shame, overwhelm) that can arise when confronted with one's complicity in systems of oppression—viewing this as a reason to respond with defensiveness, claiming futility, or leaving the work because it feels too hard, as opposed to expecting that uprooting these systems within ourselves can feel deeply uncomfortable and disorienting and leaning into it	• For example, justice-oriented work centered in individual and collective healing
		• For example, centering somatics as part of this work
	• For example, can reproduce stereotypes about "the angry Black woman" when such individuals try to bring forward legitimate concerns about structure racism in healthcare	

The language of "allyship" is used:	As an identity claimed by a person in a position of privilege to elevate their status The primary motivation for the person in a position of privilege is demonstrating one's goodness; therefore, actions need to be seen and rewarded Linked to kindness, generosity, or goodness • For example, EDI efforts focused on "being an ally" • For example, EDI efforts that start with the assumption that the problem is "bad apples" who need to be stopped (e.g., racists) by good people who are the "allies" • This can manifest as a focus on individual-level microaggressions, without locating that work in the context of broader interesting systems of oppression	As a concept only from the perspective of people on the bottom of the coin The primary motivation for the person in a position of privilege is accountable and responsible action given how one is structured in history; therefore, actions are frequently unseen and resist reward Linked to radical, solidarity-oriented collective action • Better terms might include coliberator, coconspirator, or accomplice • For example, EDI efforts that start with concern for *how* (not *if*) systems of oppression are playing out in healthcare
The approach to discrimination based on social identity is that:	These issues are separate, unconnected, and in competition with each other • For example, EDI work that pits communities against each other ("oppression Olympics") • For example, addressing the needs of people with disabilities by advocating for attention and funding over other communities (e.g., in competition with Black health, or trans healthcare, without recognizing that disabled people can also be Black and trans)	These systems of inequality are interconnected, interlocking, and mutually reinforcing • For example, EDI work oriented to a coherent intersectional power analysis • Recognizes the divide and conquer logic as a tactic for upholding oppression • For example, addressing the needs of people with disability through the lens of "disability justice," which centers the leadership of Indigenous, Black, and racialized and queer/trans disability leaders ("10 Principles of Disability Justice" 2015)

continued

Table 3.1 *continued*

	Entrenching the status quo	Toward transformation
The place of whiteness as a power structure is:	Irrelevant, unnamed, unwelcome in the room	Central to all analysis, understood as being at the core of colonization and racism, which gives rise to the other systems of inequality
	• For example, EDI committees that are deeply concerned with justice but without ever naming, recognizing, or calling into question the ways that whiteness as a power structure plays out not only in healthcare but also in EDI efforts	Includes a deep concern with *proximity to* whiteness
	• For example, action on accessibility in healthcare that does not also call into question the ways some approaches to addressing ableism uphold the power structure of whiteness	• For example, taking lessons from the "disability justice" movement in terms of a justice movement reflecting critically on its own complicity in upholding other systems of oppression (Reynolds 2022)
	• Questioning the power structure of whiteness is equated with assigning all White people as bad	

[a]Ideas in this table were inspired in part by the work by K. E. Edwards, 2006. "Aspiring Social Justice Ally Identity Development: A Conceptual Model," *NASPA Journal* 43 (4): 39–60.

disadvantage. This outcome is not an accident—the systems of oppression are working as they were designed. The result is real danger to our patients, clients, families, friends, and communities when our actions (knowingly and unknowingly) allow these systems of oppression to continue.

Table 3.1 attempts to illustrate how antioppressive approaches might lead to transformational change. This shift in orientation translates to explicit shifts in power by acknowledging the existence of systems of oppression, reframing assumptions about expertise, and accordingly, redistributing resources and control. For the coins where we find ourselves on top, we are called to actively unlearn that we are the default experts on how to dismantle systems of oppression in healthcare and that the goal is to *help* marginalized people. This reorientation allows the focus to be on the real problem, intersecting systems of oppression, and how they operate to produce exclusion, inequity, and harm throughout healthcare.

Antioppressive practice (which might also be framed as practicing critical allyship or being a coliberator) is not a linear journey, nor is it a simple transition from one thing to another. It is an active, messy process that requires constant critical reflection and a big dose of humility.

As authors who strive to be in the practice of this work, we note that our actions in healthcare do not happen only in the "toward transformation" column. Too often we find ourselves falling back into actions aligned with "entrenching the status quo." Reorienting ourselves is an ongoing practice that foregrounds the importance of nurturing a community of people who understand and are actively engaged in antioppressive practice. We ask ourselves:

> Who are the people we have gathered around us who can both provide us with care during this fraught and messy practice and also lovingly hold us to account when we slip into the middle column?
> Who are yours?

References

Sins Invalid. 2015. "10 Principles of Disability Justice." 2015. September 17. https://www.sinsinvalid.org/blog/10-principles-of-disability-justice.

Aqil, Anushka R., Mannat Malik, Keilah A. Jacques, Krystal Lee, Lauren J. Parker, Caitlin E. Kennedy, Graham Mooney, and Danielle German. 2021. "Engaging in Anti-Oppressive Public Health Teaching: Challenges and Recommendations." *Pedagogy in Health Promotion* 7 (4): 344–353.

Atewologun, Doyin. 2018. "Intersectionality Theory and Practice." In *Oxford Research Encyclopedias, Business and Management*. Oxford University Press. 10.1093/acrefore/9780190224851.013.48

Crenshaw, Kimberlé Williams. 2002. "Mapping the Margins: Intersectionality, Identity Politics, and Violence against Women of Color." In *An Introduction to Women's Studies: Gender in a Transnational World*, edited by Grewal Inderpal Kaplan Caren, 207–213. McGraw Hill.

Dougherty, Geoff B., Sherita H. Golden, Alden L. Gross, Elizabeth Colantuoni, and Lorraine T. Dean. 2020. "Measuring Structural Racism and Its Association With BMI." *American Journal of Preventive Medicine* 59 (4): 530–537.

Galloway, Mollie K., Petra Callin, Shay James, Harriette Vimegnon, and Lisa McCall. 2019. "Culturally Responsive, Antiracist, or Anti-Oppressive? How Language Matters for School Change Efforts." *Equity & Excellence in Education: University of Massachusetts School of Education Journal* 52 (4): 485–501.

Harlow, Elizabeth, and Jeff Hearn. 1996. "Educating for Anti-Oppressive and Anti-Discriminatory Social Work Practice." *Social Work in Education* 15 (1): 5–17.

Kumashiro, Kevin K. 2000. "Toward a Theory of Anti-Oppressive Education." *Review of Educational Research* 70 (1): 25–53.

Lavallee, B. and Harding, L. 2022. "Chapter 4: How Indigenous-specific Racism is Coached into Health Systems". In *White Benevolence: Racism and Colonial Violence in the Helping Professions*, edited by Amanda Gebhard, Sheelah McLean and Verna St. Denis. Halifax: Fernwood Publishing.

Lavallée, L. F. 2014. "Anti-Oppression Research." In *The SAGE Encyclopedia of Action Research*, edited by David Coghlan and Mary Brydon-Miller, 1:40–44. SAGE Publications.

Lukachko, Alicia, Mark L. Hatzenbuehler, and Katherine M. Keyes. 2014. "Structural Racism and Myocardial Infarction in the United States." *Social Science & Medicine* 103 (February): 42–50.

Lyons, Vivian H., Jessie Seiler, Ali Rowhani-Rahbar, and Avanti Adhia. 2023. "Lessons Learned from Integrating Anti-Oppression Pedagogy in a Graduate-Level Course in Epidemiology." *American Journal of Epidemiology* 192 (8): 1231–1237.

McIntosh, P. 1988. "White Privilege and Male Privilege: A Personal Account of Coming to See Correspondences through Work in Women's Studies." Working paper no. 189. http://www.nationalseedproject.org/images/documents/White_Privilege_and_Male_Privilege_Personal_Account-Peggy_McIntosh.pdf.

Morgan, Kathryn Pauly. 1996. "Describing the Emperor's New Clothes: Three Myths of Educational (In)Equality." In *The Gender Question in Education: Theory, Pedagogy and Politics*, edited by Ann Diller, Barbara Houston, Kathryn Pauly Morgan, and Maryann Ayim, 272. Westview.

Nixon, Stephanie. 2020. "Understanding the Role of Privilege in Relation to Public Health Ethics and Practice." YouTube. Posted October 6, 2020. https://www.youtube.com/watch?v=a30a_NiT5zc&list=PLNWUsONW1NHKByYnDkqHAFpoCXcGuIGa4&index=5.

Nixon, Stephanie. 2021. *Tips for Effective Allyship*. Vimeo. https://vimeo.com/644652449.

Nixon, Stephanie A. 2019. "The Coin Model of Privilege and Critical Allyship: Implications for Health." *BMC Public Health* 19 (1): 1637.

Reynolds, Joel Michael. 2022. "Disability and White supremacy." *Critical Philosophy of Race* 10 (1): 48–70.

Wallace, Maeve, Joia Crear-Perry, Lisa Richardson, Meshawn Tarver, and Katherine Theall. 2017. "Separate and Unequal: Structural Racism and Infant Mortality in the US." *Health & Place* 45 (May): 140–144.

Zinga, Dawn, and Sandra Styres. 2019. "Decolonizing Curriculum: Student Resistances to Anti-Oppressive Pedagogy." *Power and Education* 11 (1): 30–50.

Chapter 4
Health Equity Frameworks for Structural and Behavioral Change

Sherrie Flynt-Wallington

Introduction

You may see the terms "health disparities" and "health equity" used in various contexts such that you may believe these terms mean the same thing; however, they are not interchangeable. They are two distinct constructs that should be defined and operationalized as such. In an early 2014 article on health disparities and health equity, Paula Braveman calls on researchers to be clear and highlights the importance of specifying the definition of "health disparity" and "health equity" to ensure their intended purposes: identifying differences in health due to more specific disadvantages. Healthy People 2020 defined "health disparities" as health differences due to social, economic, and environmental disadvantages, which helped shift the term from general health differences to, more specifically, health differences due to injustices(cite?). This definition also specifically emphasizes how these health differences affect particular people who have faced additional obstacles based on "their racial or ethnic group, religion, socioeconomic status, gender, age, or mental health; cognitive, sensory, or physical disability; sexual orientation or gender identity; geographic location; or other characteristics historically linked to discrimination or exclusion" (Braveman 2014).

As defined by the Centers for Disease Control and Prevention (CDC), health equity is "the state in which everyone has a fair and just opportunity to attain their highest level of health" (Office of Heallth Equity 2024). Achieving health equity is a commitment to eliminate the health disparities that exist today (Braveman 2014). Health disparities come from preventable differences in the way individuals suffer from disease, injury, or violence due to their racial/ethnic, socioeconomic, and/or environmental differences (Office of Health Equity 2024). These disparities have often come from

Sherrie Flynt-Wallington, *Health Equity Frameworks for Structural and Behavioral Change*. In: *Power, Privilege, and Public Health in the United States*. Edited by: Lorraine T. Dean and Keilah A. Jacques, Oxford University Press.
© Oxford University Press (2025). DOI: 10.1093/9780197760956.003.0004

generational injustices that have been systemically implanted into policies, practices, and explicit and implicit bias that continuously cause preventable hardship for vulnerable populations (George Washington University Milken Institute School of Public Health 2020).

The difference between health equity and health equality lies in the accessibility of just healthcare to all. Health equality ensures that people are given the same resources or opportunities regardless of their current social, financial, educational, or geographical situation, which could also involve health disparities (George Washington University Milken Institute School of Public Health 2020). Social determinants of health (SODH) are key identifiable differences that help explain health disparities and how they develop and affect individuals. There are five domains within social determinants of health: (1) economic stability, (2) educational access and quality, (3) healthcare access and quality, (4) neighborhood and built environment, and (5) social and community context (US Department of Health and Human Services n.d.). These domains help explain differences in how people live and where health disparities exist, which in turn affect their opportunities to obtain the highest level of health, even with equal resources or opportunities.

As defined by the Pan American Health Organization, health equity is "a fundamental component of social justice that indicates the absence of avoidable, unfair or remediable differences among groups of people due to their social, economic, demographic or geographic circumstances" (Pan American Health Organization n.d.). Social determinants of health have aided researchers and public health departments uncover how to effectively target these existing inequities and injustices and supply information to support needed change to achieve healthcare equity (Narain and Zimmerman 2018).

Emergence of the Terms "Health Disparities" and "Health Equity"

A search for the term "health disparities" in the electronic database PubMed returned 105,539 results. These results were filtered by publication date and the phrase "health disparity and health equity." The first article listed was published in 1965 in *The New England Journal of Medicine*. This article's summary referenced Public Law 88.156, signed by President Kennedy on October 24, 1963, which shifted focus on the need for greater maternal and child health services (Anderson et al. 1965). The article discusses findings related to an increased frequency of intellectual disabilities and other impairments found in those with "inadequate maternal and child health services,"

(Anderson et al. 1965). This early article is a recognition of health disparities starting to emerge among unique populations related to differences in health services received.

Additionally, in the search results for "health disparities," the word "inequities" starts to emerge in the titles of articles as well as in the article abstracts or summaries. One example is a 1982 article titled "Black Health Inequities and the American Health Care System," in which the abstract states, "This paper examines the health care status of blacks in the American health care system and points out that blacks are burdened by a number of health inequities when compared to their white counterparts" (Rice and Jones 1982). Looking deeper at the search results, the terms "inequities" and "health inequities" appear more often than "disparities" among the titles in works published between 1965 and the 1990s. The search results from the 1990s frequently include the terms "disparities," "socioeconomical disparities," "racial disparities," and "health disparities," in addition to "inequities."

The search for "health equity" in the PubMed database returned 55,834 results. The first article listed was from 1970, titled "Community Participation for Equity and Excellence in Health Care. General Discussion I." The publication is a discussion from the 1970 Health Conference of the New York Academy of Medicine, which shared ideas to provide healthcare services to all who need them (Community Participation for Equity and Excellence in Health Care 1970).

The search results for both "health disparities" and "health equity" show a significant increase in published articles at the start of the 1980s and show a steady and steep increase in search results in the 1990s and early 2000s. A significant event included in the CDC's "Achievements and Milestones in CDC's Efforts to 'Bake In' Health Equity," was the release of "The Report of the Secretary's Task Force on Black and Minority Health." The report was released in 1985 and discusses the "existence of health disparities among racial and ethnic minorities in the United States" (Office of Health Equity 2024). The release of this report correlates with the increase in published articles listed when searching for the key terms "health disparities" and "health equity."

Theoretical Framework and Approaches

The use of "health equity" and "health disparity" and their increasing frequency can be linked to their emergence in the literature. However, as actual constructs or concepts, each term is complex and requires varied theoretical lenses and approaches to better understand each phrase's impact on population health. Several frameworks and approaches guide the development of social determinants of health (SDOH) research. These frameworks build upon the concept of the "social gradient"—that individuals with lower social status have greater health risks and lower life expectancy than those with higher status and that the impact of social position can accumulate over time (Marmot and Bell 2016). Earlier research by Marmot et al. (2008) suggested that observed differences in social determinants are thought to develop from unequal distribution of resources; thus, they can be reduced through targeted social and economic policies and programs. A few of these have garnered a lot of attention due to their wide use and because they address multilevel aspects of disparities and health equity.

Though this is not an exhaustive list, the following frameworks provide a unique contribution of theoretical frameworks and approaches that may provide an explanatory lens for understanding disparities and collectively provide a much-needed structured foundation for investigating disparities and health equity.

Social-Ecological Model

The social-ecological model (SEM) describes the layers of influence on individual health behavior, decision-making, and actions. The Centers for Disease Control and Prevention illustrate this model (2024) as a series of nested rings, with the individual at the center (micro). The next layer of influence refers to the individual's immediate social circle, interpersonal, followed by organizational (work or school environments) and then community (messo); finally, society (macro) is the outermost ring. SEM is a powerful structure for understanding how various influences impact individual health, illustrating how bigger influences impact populations one individual at a time. For example, communities often experience health disparities due to community-wide factors.

A recent study exploring older adults' perceptions of and comfort with walking in their community, a significant health-related mechanism, utilized SEM to structure the study and propose future research in the area (Leung et al. 2021). SEM also provided structure for understanding the themes that emerged from the research—individual benefits and barriers, interpersonal social support and norms, community environment (e.g., benches, sidewalks, shade, traffic), and policy/societal factors (cultural norms and policies that impact walkability). The recommended interventions also corresponded to concrete, impactful actions at each of the model levels.

Structural Influence Model of Health Communication

The structural influence model of health communication (SIM) states that social determinants of health—the factors of where individuals live, work, and learn that impact their individual and community health and thereby health inequity—influence communication outcomes (Viswanath et al. 2007). These outcomes can include the capacity to access, process, and respond to communication messages which can lead to adverse health outcomes and disparities. SIM provides a model for understanding the relationship between the social determinants of health and communication outcomes.

In response to health communication challenges throughout the early stages of the COVID-19 pandemic, one study utilized SIM to understand the exacerbated disparities and to identify considerations in health communications to improve health outcomes (Häfliger et al. 2023). Häfliger et al. found a primarily lower education level to be studied as a factor impacting communication outcomes, suggesting (1) that health communication messages need to effectively target people with lower educational levels and (2) that research is needed on how communication inequalities and health disparities impact groups of people with vulnerable immigration status, financial hardship, language challenges; gender and sexual minorities; and racial and ethnic minorities. They also recommend that future research be conducted to assess communication strategies for impacting health disparities in public health crises.

Community-Based Participatory Research

Community-based participatory research (CBPR) is similar to patient-centered communication in a clinical setting for public health research. CBPR is based on an equal relationship between researchers and community partners, starting with the initial study design and priority setting and continuing throughout the research and through the dissemination of the findings (Israel et al. 2010). CBPR builds community capacity and aims for positive long-term relationships between researchers and community members. As a result, CBPR is an ideal research model for addressing health disparities and focusses on many traditional barriers to community partnerships and community-based interventions.

One excellent example of CBPR having a long-term impact on health disparities is an intervention in Atlanta, Georgia, which developed a care coordination program for underserved, high-risk patients (Williams-Livingston et al. 2020). Through collaboration with community stakeholders and researchers, it was determined that a patient-centered medical home was needed. A neighborhood-based pilot intervention was developed and successfully deployed. The lessons learned from the pilot program will be used to train clinicians and practices.

Another example of CBPR in action is the study Reach Out churches, where University of Michigan and Eastern Michigan University academic partners collaborated with community partners from Bridges into the Future, a faith-based organization in Flint, Michigan, to address hypertension and prevention among members of local faith-based organizations (Skolarus et al. 2018). Academic and community partners met weekly and collaborated on choosing the health prevention focus throughout each phase of the process. Recruitment through the faith-based organizations, because of the trust and rapport developed over time before the intervention, was positive; the structure and tone of the intervention (text message communication for tracking blood pressure) was found largely acceptable among participants, and trust in the randomization process, due to trust in the partners running the intervention, was relatively high. Other research attempts in similar demographics (majority African American, low-income communities) have often been less successful without the relationship-building that is the foundation of CBPR.

Intersectionality Framework

Intersectionality (or intersectional theory) is a term first coined in 1989 by American civil rights advocate and leading scholar of critical race theory Kimberlé Williams Crenshaw (2017). It focuses on intersecting social identities and related systems of oppression, domination, or discrimination. As an analytical framework, intersectionality seeks to understand how individuals' various social and political identities result in unique combinations of discrimination and privilege. The framework serves as a lens for six core ideas: social inequality, power relations, relationality, social context, complexity, and social justice (Collins 2022).

The intersectionality framework has been used to examine racial/ethnic minorities at risk of and living with HIV and often possessing multiple stigmas (e.g., HIV-positive, substance use) (Earnshaw et al. 2013). More recent and fascinating work focuses on the use of the intersectionality framework and surgical disparities. Chen et al. (2022) propose a more inclusive approach that incorporates the interaction of multiple marginalized identities with social determinants of health and its implications on surgical outcomes. Chapter 6 of this book is devoted to a full explication of intersectionality theory.

Active Community Engagement Continuum

The active community engagement continuum (ACE) is a conceptual framework of three levels of engagement across five characteristics of community engagement (community involvement in assessment, access to information, inclusion in decision-making, community capacity to advocate for needs, and accountability of institutions to the community; Russell et al. 2008). Level 1 describes a basic community-based model, where the decision-making and power are largely maintained by academic or government institutions in which community involvement is more superficial. Level 2 describes research and interventions that involve collaboration with community members. Level 3 describes equitable participation in all levels of decision-making and priority-setting with community partners. The ACE is a tool for measuring current or past collaboration and a model for planning future collaboration.

The ACQUIRE Project, a reproductive health access project, developed and utilized the continuum to analyze family planning and reproductive health interventions internationally based on their level of community engagement, as well as to plan and execute long-lasting change interventions through community engagement. The structured continuum also provided a common reference for community and academic partners to discuss their preferred level of collaboration (Russell et al. 2008).

National Institute on Minority Health and Health Disparities Research Framework

The National Institute on Minority Health and Health Disparities (NIMHD) Research Framework (2017) was developed to encourage research that addresses the complex nature of health disparities, including interdisciplinary research across levels of influence (from SEM). The framework provides a structure for classifying that facilitates analysis of research regarding health disparities (National Institute on Minority Health and Health Disparities [NIMHD] 2017). The framework is a grid that spans domains of influence—biological, behavioral, physical/built environment, sociocultural environment, and healthcare system. Those domains are looked at in relation to the levels of influence from SEM—individual, interpersonal, community, and societal—and outcomes at each level.

One example of the application of the NIMHD Framework involves reexamining the continuum from fundamental access to healthcare (including insurance-based discrimination) to the patient-centered medical home (PCMH) model through the lens of patient engagement and empowerment (Spencer and Chen 2023). The framework follows various experiences—from not being able to access care or find a provider willing to take Medicare (which reimburses at substantially lower rates than private insurance or Medicaid), through various models of patient-provider communication, to the proverbial pinnacle model of PCMH. By seeing these experiences on the same plane, we see the concrete mechanisms of discrimination becoming health outcomes, and it provides the opportunity to recommend a variety of actions for impact at various levels of influence.

In particular, the emphasis on community-engaged and intersectionality approaches stresses the need for authentic collaboration, equitable power, and resources. Communities must be respected for the value of their subject matter expertise and their perceived priorities, specifically, health priorities for themselves and their communities. Communities must be involved in the matters that will impact them in order for the identification and implementation of actionable and equitable solutions for sustained change to take place regarding disparity reduction and the achievement of health equity. This, along with the recognition of the importance and complexities of intersectionality (Crenshaw 2017), which speaks to race and gender as well as the range of "social categories" such as disability, sexual orientation, occupation, and socioeconomic disadvantage, are important in understanding the factors that promote and impede health equity.

Social Determinants of Health

Operationalizing the specific definitions through the lens of these frameworks also creates a clearer understanding of the important social determinants of health and mechanisms that are at play in relation to disparities and health equity. These include social factors, upstream and downstream factors, life course factors, pathways and biological mechanisms, global data gaps, and lack of political will.

Social Factors

A critical body of SDOH explores pathways including social and biological mechanisms and provides a previously unavailable scientific foundation that appreciates the fundamental role of social and structural factors in health (Braveman et al. 2011). Research has long established that social factors are important influences on health (Braveman et al. 2011; Braveman and Gottlieb 2014; Palmer et al. 2019). We must now move beyond that to address how social factors operate and how we can most effectively intervene to activate health-promoting pathways and interrupt health-damaging ones.

Upstream and Downstream Factors

Little attention has been given to upstream SDOH (i.e., economic resources, education, and racial discrimination). These upstream determinants represent the fundamental causes in pathways that influence downstream factors and ultimately lead to health effects (Braveman and Gottlieb 2014; Sheingold et al. 2023). One barrier to understanding how upstream social determinants influence health is a widespread expectation that a single research study can encompass an entire pathway—from upstream factors to downstream health effects. Such studies are unlikely to be effective due to the complex causal chains and prolonged periods involved. Instead, research should focus on advancing knowledge of pathways incrementally by linking results from studies of specific pathway segments.

Life Course Factors

Individual and population health risks arise from multiple sources across the life course. Risk factors and adverse exposures are found in multiple domains and often cluster in socially patterned ways that synergistically influence short- and long-term consequences (Hertzman and Boyce 2010; Jones et al. 2019). Most research designs characterize effects on health outcomes of single exposures and rarely assess the importance of the timing of exposures or influences over time (e.g., over a life course; Jones et al. 2019; Kuh et al. 2003). Life course perspectives on health disparities propose that socially patterned environmental exposures influence the development of biological, physiological, and psychosocial systems, including structural and functional changes in the brain. Developmental and structural perspectives on the life course arise from distinct theories that warrant closer integration into research on how biological mechanisms result in health disparities (Jones et al. 2019).

Equally important is the current siloed approach to research (e.g., biological, psychological, sociological, environmental, anthropological, and population health). Segmentation into disease focus and fragmented healthcare delivery foci may limit the ability to integrate SDOH life course concepts and frameworks, models, and approaches to advance SDOH research more broadly and effectively. Increasing and supporting interdisciplinary research, although rewarding and offering the potential for high yield, requires understanding the significant level of effort required to blend disciplines, expertise, and methodology (Jones et al. 2019).

Pathways and Biological Mechanisms

Evidence demonstrates that the chronic stress of social disadvantage, socioeconomic inequality, and racial discrimination works through a variety of biological pathways to influence health, including neuroendocrine, developmental, immunologic, and vascular mechanisms (Braveman et al. 2011; Wolfe and Evans 2012). More research on pathways and biological mechanisms is needed, as are well-designed studies of interventions. Challenges to designing and adequately studying multidimensional interventions that simultaneously address multiple factors remain and have long been discussed (Braveman and Gottlieb 2014; Marmot et al. 2008; Thimm-Kaiser et al. 2023).

Specific research related to cellular signaling that links known associations between SDOH, chronic stress, and adversity to certain chronic health diseases is also lacking. There is an absence of data surrounding what is currently known about these associations and signaling pathways downstream of psychosocial and environmental stress. Other focal areas of interest are epigenetic regulation of the chronic stress response and the effects of SDOH on telomere length and aging (Baumer et al. 2023; Notterman and Mitchell 2015).

Global Data Gaps: A Data Conundrum

There are substantial global data gaps across contexts and different dimensions related to SDOH (Biermann et al. 2021). Data on SDOH vary in availability (e.g., in low-income settings), ownership (e.g., public versus private), comprehensiveness of sources (e.g., insufficient population-based sources such as vital registration, census, and surveys), types (e.g., qualitative and quantitative), and levels of data (e.g., national versus local). This lack of data stagnates SDOH research and demonstrates the importance of analyzing and understanding SDOH relative to the contexts in which they are experienced (Biermann et al. 2021; Office of the High Commissioner 2018). Biermann et al. (2021) and other global organizations suggest that data use is challenged by the complexity and interconnectedness of SDOH that call for integrated and intersectoral approaches to tackle health outcomes. Researchers should push data collection, and disaggregation must go beyond gender, geography, and age to ensure that all health determinants are identified and addressed to leave no one behind (Lopez and Gadsden 2016). Simply put, context does matter. The context—global, national, or local—may also determine which SDOHs are the priorities that impact strategies, policy and funding, and overall political will (Post et al. 2010).

Lack of Political Will

Despite growing evidence on SDOH and important linkages to health equity, political action has not been as robust as the actual research. Political will is most simply defined as "the extent of committed support among key decision-makers for a particular policy solution to a particular problem" (Post et al. 2010). Little is known about how political will operates to enact equity promoting policies. A lack of political will is seen as a crucial barrier to advancing actionable SDOH solutions and research.

A strategic research agenda on SDOH should also address factors that can (1) enhance or impede political will to translate knowledge into effective action, (2) determine how path dependency that exacerbates health inequities can be broken, (3) explore working with sympathetic political forces committed to fairness, (4) frame policy options in a way that makes them more likely to be adopted, (5) outline factors to consider in challenging the interests of elites, and (6) consider the extent to which civil society will work in favor of equitable policies (Baum et al. 2022; Finnemore and Sikkink 1998; Knight et al. 2012). These data gaps, along with the thin line of research, hinder the ability to comprehend how SDOH informs policymaking to reduce disparities and achieve health equity.

Taken together, how we language, define, and operationalize health disparities and health hold significant weight. More importantly, our theoretical frameworks and approaches, particularly those approaches that integrate diverse voices from individuals and communities, are how we will eventually get to actionable changes in health disparities and achieve health equity. From this and the other chapters, we see that disparities are multilayered and complex. Understanding the important mechanisms helps us to better understand the factors that drive the social determinants and how and when we can intervene.

References

Anderson, Ursula M., Rachel Jenss, William E. Mosher, Clyde L. Randall, and Edward Marra. 1965. "High-Risk Groups: Definition and Identification." *New England Journal of Medicine* 273 (6): 308–313.

Baum, Fran, Belinda Townsend, Matt Fisher, Kathryn Browne-Yung, Toby Freeman, Anna Ziersch, Patrick Harris, and Sharon Friel. 2022. "Creating Political Will for Action on Health Equity: Practical Lessons for Public Health Policy Actors." *International Journal of Health Policy and Management* 11 (7): 947.

Baumer, Yvonne, Mario A. Pita, Andrew S. Baez, Lola R. Ortiz-Whittingham, Manuel A. Cintron, Rebecca R. Rose, Veronica C. Gray, Foster Osei Baah, and Tiffany M. Powell-Wiley. 2023. "By What Molecular Mechanisms Do Social Determinants Impact Cardiometabolic Risk?" *Clinical Science* 137 (6): 469–494.

Biermann, Olivia, Meggie Mwoka, Catherine K. Ettman, Salma M. Abdalla, Sherine Shawky, Jane Ambuko, Mark Pearson, et al. 2021. "Data, Social Determinants, and Better Decision-Making for Health: The 3-D Commission." *Journal of Urban Health* 98 (Suppl 1): 4–14.

Braveman, Paula, Susan Egerter, and David Williams. 2011. "The Social Determinants of Health: Coming of Age." *Review of Public Health* 32: 381–398.

Braveman, Paula. 2014. "What Are Health Disparities and Health Equity? We Need to Be Clear." *Public Health Reports* 129 (1, Suppl 2): 5–8.

Braveman, Paula, and Laura Gottlieb. 2014. "The Social Determinants of Health: It's Time to Consider the Causes of the Causes." *Public Health Reports* 129 (1, Suppl 2): 19–31.

Chen, J. C., and Samilia Obeng-Gyasi. 2022. "Intersectionality and the Surgical Patient: Expanding the Surgical Disparities Framework." *Annals of Surgery* 275 (1): e3–e5.

Collins, Patricia Hill. 2022. *Black Feminist Thought: Knowledge, Consciousness, and the Politics of Empowerment*. Routledge.

Cordice, John W. V. Jr. 1970. "Community participation for equity and excellence in health care. General discussion IV". *Bulletin of the New York Academy of Medicine* 46 (12): 1149–1150.

Crenshaw, Kimberlé. 2017. *On Intersectionality: Essential Writings.* New York: The New Press.

Earnshaw, Valerie A., Laura M. Bogart, John F. Dovidio, and David R. Williams. 2015. "Stigma and Racial/Ethnic HIV Disparities: Moving toward Resilience." *The American Psychologist* 68 (4): 225–236.

Earnshaw, V. A., L. R., Smith, S. R., Chaudoir, K. R., Amico, and M. M. Copenhaver, M.M. 2013. "HIV Stigma Mechanisms and Well-beign amoung PLWH: a Test of the HIV Stigma Framework." *Aids and Behavior* 17 (5): 1785–1795.

Finnemore, Martha, and Kathryn Sikkink. 1998. "International Norm Dynamics and Political Change." *International Organization* 52 (4): 887–917.

George Washington University Milken Institute School of Public Health. 2020. "Online Public Health Resources: Equity vs. Equality: What's the Difference?" https://onlinepublichealth.gwu.edu/resources/equity-vs-equality/.

Häfliger, Clara, Nicola Diviani, and Sara Rubinelli. 2023. "Communication Inequalities and Health Disparities among Vulnerable Groups during the COVID-19 Pandemic: A Scoping Review of Qualitative and Quantitative Evidence." *BMC Public Health* 23 (1): 428.

Hertzman, Clyde, and Tom Boyce. 2010. "How Experience Gets under the Skin to Create Gradients in Developmental Health." *Annual Review of Public Health* 31: 329–347.

Israel, Barbara A., Chris M. Coombe, Rebecca R. Cheezum, Amy J. Schulz, Robert J. McGranaghan, Richard Lichtenstein, Angela G. Reyes, Jaye Clement, and Akosua Burris. 2010. "Community-Based Participatory Research: A Capacity-Building Approach for Policy Advocacy Aimed at Eliminating Health Disparities." *American Journal of Public Health* 100 (11): 2094–2102.

Jones, Neal L., Sarah E. Gilman, Tina L. Cheng, Steven S. Drury, Catherine V. Hill, and Arline T. Geronimus. 2019. "Life Course Approaches to the Causes of Health Disparities." *American Journal of Public Health* 109 (S1): S48–S55.

Knight, Eric. 2012. *Reframe: How to Solve the World's Trickiest Problems.* Black.

Kuh, Diana, Yoav Ben-Shlomo, Michael G. Marmot, Marcus E. Davey Smith, George Davey Smith, and Shah Ebrahim. 2003. "Life Course Epidemiology." *Journal of Epidemiology & Community Health*, 57: 778–783.

Leung, K. M., K. L. Ou, P. K. Chung, and C. Thøgersen-Ntoumani. 2021. "Older Adults' Perceptions toward Walking: A Qualitative Study Using a Social-Ecological Model." *International Journal of Environmental Research and Public Health* 18 (14): 7686.

López, Nancy, and Vivian Gadsen. 2016. "Health Inequities, Social Determinants, and Intersectionality." December 5, 2016. https://nam.edu/health-inequities-social-determinants-and-intersectionality/.

Marmot, M., R. Bell. 2016. "Social Inequalities in Health: a Proper Concern of Epidemiology." *Annals of Epidemiology* 26 (4): 238–240.

Marmot, M., S. Friel, R. Bell, T. A. Houweling, S. Taylor, and Commission on Social Determinants of Health. 2008. "Closing the Gap in a Generation: Health Equity through Action on the Social Determinants of Health." *Lancet* 372 (9650): 1661–1669.

Narain, K., and F. Zimmerman. 2018. "Advancing Health Equity: Facilitating Action on the Social Determinants of Health among Public Health Departments." *American Journal of Public Health* 108 (6): 737–738.

National Institute on Minority Health and Health Disparities. 2017. "NIMHD Research Framework." Accessed December 2, 2023. https://nimhd.nih.gov/researchFramework.

Notterman, D. A., and C. Mitchell. 2015. "Epigenetics and Understanding the Impact of Social Determinants of Health." *Pediatric Clinics of North America* 62 (5): 1227–1240.

Office of Health Equity. 2024. "What Is Health Equity?" Centers for Disease Control and Prevention. https://www.cdc.gov/healthequity/whatis/index.html.

Office of the High Commissioner (OHCHR). 2018. "*A Human Rights-Based Approach to Data. Leaving No One Behind in the 2030 Agenda for Sustainable Development.*" United Nations Human Rights Office of the High Commissioner.

Palmer, R. C., D. Ismond, E. J. Rodriquez, and J. S. Kaufman. 2019. "Social Determinants of Health: Future Directions for Health Disparities Research." *American Journal of Public Health* 109 (S1): S70–S71.

Pan American Health Organization. N.d. "Health Equity." Accessed November 29, 2023. https://www.paho.org/en/topics/health-equity#:~:text=Health%20Equity%20is%20a%20fundamental,economic%2C%20demographic%20or%20geographic%20circumstances.Post.

Post, Lori Ann, Amber N. W. Raile, and Eric D. Raile. 2010. "Defining Political Will." *Political Policy* 38 (4): 653–676.

Rice M. F., W. Jones Jr. 1982. "Black health inequities and the American health care system." *Health Policy Education* 10 (3):195–214.

Russell, Nancy, Susan Igras, Nalin Johri, Henrietta Kuoh, Melinda Pavin, Jane Wickstrom, and The ACQUIRE Project. 2008. "The Active Community Engagement Continuum." ACQUIRE Project working paper. Accessed December 2, 2023. https://pdf.usaid.gov/pdf_docs/pnadm497.pdf.

Skolarus, L. E., J. Cowdery, M. Dome, S. Bailey, J. Baek, J. B. Byrd, S. E. Hartley, et al. 2018. "Reach Out Churches: A Community-Based Participatory Research Pilot Trial to Assess the Feasibility of a Mobile Health Technology Intervention to Reduce Blood Pressure Among African Americans." *Health Promotion Practice* 19 (4): 495–505

Sheingold, S. H., R. B. Zuckerman, N. Lew, and A. Chappel. 2023. "Social Determinants of Health, Quality of Public Health Data, and Health Equity in the United States." *American Journal of Public Health* 113 (12): 1301–1308.

Spencer, M. R. T., and J. Chen. 2023. "Revisiting Patient Engagement and Empowerment within the NIMHD Health Disparity Framework." *American Journal of Public Health* 113 (2): 141–143.

Thimm-Kaiser, M., A. Benzekri, and V. Guilamo-Ramos. 2023. "Conceptualizing the Mechanisms of Social Determinants of Health: A Heuristic Framework to Inform Future Directions for Mitigation." *Milbank Quarterly* 101 (2): 486–526.

US Department of Health and Human Services. n.d. "Healthy People 2030: Social Determinants of Health." Accessed November 29, 2023. https://health.gov/healthypeople/priority-areas/social-determinants-health.

Viswanath, K., S. Ramanadhan, and E. Z. Kontos. 2007. "Mass Media." In *Macrosocial Determinants of Population Health*, edited by S. Galea, 275–295. Springer.

Williams-Livingston, A., T. Henry Akintobi, and A. Banerjee. 2020. "Community-Based Participatory Research in Action: The Patient-Centered Medical Home and Neighborhood." *Journal of Primary Care & Community Health* 11: 2150132720968456. https://doi.org/10.1177/2150132720968456.

Wolfe, B., and W. Evans. 2012. "The Biological Consequences of Socioeconomic Inequalities." In *Social Neuroscience: Toward Understanding the Underpinnings of the Social Mind*, edited by T. E. Seeman, 1–272. Russell Sage Foundation.

Chapter 5
Guiding Principles for Conducting Research with a Health Equity Lens

Darrell Hudson

Introduction

The concept of health equity implies that everyone should be able to obtain the highest level of health possible and should not be disadvantaged because of their social position or other socially determined circumstances (Whitehead et al. 2000). Inequities in health are driven by historical policies and practices that have placed some groups at greater disadvantage relative to others (Braveman 2006). Striving toward equity requires multilevel and multisector solutions that can ameliorate past harms and contemporary barriers to achieve full health for historically marginalized people. Whitehead et al. (2000) argue that health equity involves creating opportunities and removing barriers to achieving the fullest health potential for all people. Health equity scholars have encouraged researchers to consider the development of bold solutions that move beyond proximal risk factors or individual-level health behaviors (Link and Phelan 1995; Rose 2001; Syme 2008). Centering equity in research means that scholars must contemplate equity at each stage of the research process, ranging from the ideation phase to dissemination. The goal of this chapter is to provide a broad overview of using an equity lens throughout each phase of the research process, with an emphasis on human subjects and interventional research.

Getting Started

Many different fields contribute to the advancement of health equity. Some scholars focus on delineating the myriad, impactful ways that historical legacies of racism affect contemporary health inequities. Some practitioners

Darrell Hudson, *Guiding Principles for Conducting Research with a Health Equity Lens*. In: *Power, Privilege, and Public Health in the United States*. Edited by: Lorraine T. Dean and Keilah A. Jacques, Oxford University Press.
© Oxford University Press (2025). DOI: 10.1093/9780197760956.003.0005

develop interventions to address social determinants of health or provide tailored health promotion activities to intervene in a specific health outcome. No matter what your discipline and methodological approach, if you are a health equity researcher and you want to develop a project that centers equity, the first step is often to consider what your interests and expertise are and then attempt to find a funding mechanism that would support these interests. This search for funding support could include a foundation or federal grant, in which case you are pouring over the details of a specific call or figuring the best way to align your work with the priorities outlined (Syme 2005). However, what if we have that backwards? If we are interested in addressing inequities, it seems that a key perspective would be to center the voices of those who suffer most from social, economic, and health inequities (Ford and Airhihenbuwa 2010).

The development of solutions that are truly centered on equity often require meaningful community engagement (Goodman and Sanders Thompson 2017, 2018; Hudson et al. 2023). Although a great deal is known about the sociohistorical, economic, and political forces that have driven health inequities, the development of appropriate, effective solutions often requires first-hand knowledge drawn from people who have suffered the most from inequities (Martinez et al. 2019). This includes a proper framing of the context in which people are embedded. More and more, scholars are arguing that community engagement is an effective way to develop solutions to address health inequities (Goodman and Sanders Thompson 2017; Komaie et al. 2017). Community members are experts in their own lived experiences, and it is important to engage with partners to find out what are the most important factors to foster the resilience that people are already displaying in challenging circumstances.

It is important to engage, early and often, with community members and center the voices of those who have been historically marginalized or who bear a disproportionate burden of inequities (Goodman and Sanders Thompson 2017). In fact, building relationships with these stakeholders usually starts long before the launch of a project. If there is not adequate time for authentic dialogue between community partners and research team members, transparency and trust can break down, threatening the sustainability of partnerships. Similarly, it is critical to allow time for feedback on the process and deliverables that any team proposes. This may even be prioritized over markers of project success (Hudson et al. 2023). If the feedback of community partners is not incorporated, the viability and long-term sustainability of a project will come into question. Beginning a new partnership requires researchers and community partners to navigate power dynamics, transparency, and misalignments across institutions.

However, starting the process of collaboration prior to working on a specific project or deliverable is often challenging, as there are not many funding mechanisms that support the development of partnerships. Furthermore, even when there is intentional engagement on the front end, the problems identified by community members might not align with the priorities of funding agencies (Syme 2008). For example, during the ideation phase of a project, community partners may identify challenges that do not align with current funding priorities or that may even stretch beyond the expertise and experience of a research team. Therefore, it is critical to be transparent with community partners about capacity and the supports available to support different types of work. It may also be necessary to develop a collective strategy to prioritize key issues and approaches so there is some mutual consensus in setting research goals.

In the art of community engagement, researchers and their partners must consider different levels of engagement, which could include activities that do not require high levels of trust and shared leadership, such as outreach activities, in contrast to those requiring deeper levels of engagement such as mutual agenda-setting and shared decision-making (et al. 2023). A first step for health equity researchers is to determine the most appropriate level of engagement. This includes an assessment of the researchers' own capacity, including time, bandwidth, and support, to engage in trust-building and the establishment of communication norms and decision-making processes (Goodman and Sanders Thompson 2017; Hudson et al. 2023). Conducting effective community-engaged work is challenging, as the expectations and incentive structure of academic institutions and funding agencies often collide with the priorities of community partners (Jagosh et al. 2012). Similarly, health equity scholars committed to community engagement must be flexible in order to incorporate the perspectives of community partners in projects that they are leading (Freire et al. 2015; Morrel-Samuels et al. 2016). We should also push institutions to change their incentive structures, such as more heavily weighting community-based research in promotion decisions, to reflect the additional time it takes.

Finding an appropriate community partner or set of partners is critical to an effective project. For researchers, especially those who are new to a community, looking for new community partners may start with the university. There may be a community engagement office that can help identify appropriate partners, categorized by neighborhood, sector, health condition, advocacy cause, and more. There are also informal connections that can be made between scholars who have worked in the community and created partnerships. These connections are invaluable, as direct referrals can help to accelerate the trust-building process. Similarly, referrals from potential community partners are also very helpful. While the process of meeting potential partners is fairly straightforward, there are several challenges to consider. Sustainable partnerships require continued connection and effort to maintain those connections. Often, collective efficacy and trust are developed through continually engaging and consistently showing up. Additionally, finding representative partners is sometimes challenging. For example, it may be easier to find potential partners when using referrals from university and community partners. However, it is critical to consider whether these partners are representative of the community that you are seeking to serve. It might be helpful to ask potential partners who else should be at the table. The people who are most affected by inequities are often the most difficult to reach, so it may require some intentional outreach and creativity to find the most representative community partners.

As important as it is to find the right partnerships and have community voices at the table, it is just as critical to ensure that community partners are able to fully engage. This requires effort from researchers to provide training, resources, and remuneration for time and expertise, so that community partners are prepared to engage in the research process to fully harness their voices and perspectives in the research that is being conducted (Komaie et al. 2017). For example, the Community Research Fellows Training (CRFT) program, started by Dr. Melody Goodman at Washington University in St. Louis, is devoted to the development of research capacity among community members (Goodman et al. 2017). Through a fifteen-week training format that includes at least forty-five hours of instruction plus independent learning, community members learn about the research process and key principles of health equity and build a base of knowledge related to the development of solutions for health inequities at a local level (Goodman et al. 2017; Goodman and Sanders Thompson 2018; Komaie et al. 2017). This program, started over ten years ago and focuses on equity and the development of reciprocal partnerships, and there are opportunities for seed funding that program participants can use to develop their own projects, which aids in sustainability, as fellows have skills and connections that go beyond the structure of the training program. As evidence of its success, fellows have maintained connections and incorporated the materials they were exposed to in the training into their positions (Goodman et al. 2017). Evaluation data indicate that the program is successful in increasing trainees' knowledge of social determinants of health and the research process.

Another program that centers equity in the research process through the development of sustainable, effective partnerships is the Interdisciplinary Research Leaders (IRL) program, a Robert Wood Johnson Foundation initiative (Gollust et al. 2022). This three-year program provides a wide range of supports to enhance academic-community partnerships. IRL builds the capacity of community partners, enhancing their ability to engage with researchers and to leverage research findings to advocate for policy changes. The program provides funding for a research project in which there is an intentional focus on the development of a sustainable partnership. This training is delivered through weekly webinars and semiannual meetings that bring together teams from all over the US to share their approach to achieving equity in their own local context (Gollust et al. 2022). These efforts not only assist in the development of community capacity to more fully participate in partnerships, but they also make the playing field more even, centering power rather than allowing academic researchers to drive directions and activities (Gollust et al. 2022; Mattessich and Johnson 2018). This includes the development of leadership skills that span different sectors and disciplines, creating a national network of partners to advance health equity. IRL seeks to foster action-oriented research that is beneficial to local communities and is ethical, accessible, and aligned with community standards. For researchers, training enhances their ability to authentically engage with community partners, to translate research into policy and practice, and to understand how the policy process works at different levels.

No matter the approach taken, it is critical to assess where you are as a researcher and/or practitioner. This includes an honest consideration of what your own biases may be in addition to your expertise. In the search for appropriate partners, it is important to consider what is the most appropriate level of engagement and whether a researcher and their team has enough resources to engage in an authentic manner (Goodman and Sanders Thompson 2017).

Theoretical Scaffolding (What's theory got to do with it?)

It is also critical to use an appropriate theoretical framework to guide equity (Carpiano and Daley 2006; Hudson 2021, 2023). Theory is important and helpful because it helps to outline and define key factors and linkages that explain a phenomenon (Carpiano and Daley 2006). Theory can help to provide conceptual clarity to define key terms, establish directionality between concepts, and provide a guide to reproduce results over time. Theory provides a roadmap to measurement and helps to guide the methodological map for the development of an approach or the eventual implementation and evaluation of a program. Theory also aids with the creation of best practices through systematization of knowledge, explanations, and predictions. In many ways, theory drives the development of a coherent evidence base through the identification and establishment of the most appropriate, effective approaches to addressing health inequities. Furthermore, theory can help to guide researchers and practitioners to examine how to engage in power mapping, identifying where power is located and where power needs to be shifted in order to strive toward equity (Hudson 2023). Whenever we describe relationships between elements, we imply theory—even if we don't explicitly state what that theory is. As scientists, working toward transparency and reproducibility of our science, it is our responsibility to explicitly state the theory we are using or testing.

It is also important to rigorously test and evaluate theory (Carpiano and Daley 2006). This is critical when applying theory with an equity lens. Applying theory with an equity lens means that researchers and practitioners must be aware of sociohistorical factors that fuel health inequities and shape the contexts in which people are embedded. For example, scholars have argued that many of the most commonly used health behavior theories do not adequately center equity (Braveman et al. 2011; Sanders Thompson 2009). Specifically, health behavior theories that primarily emphasize individual-level factors (e.g., cognitive processes, knowledge, attitudes, and beliefs) as the key drivers of health behavior without paying adequate attention to the social and environmental context in which people are embedded will have limited explanatory power and applied impact for health equity. Similarly, from a theoretical perspective, it is critical to recognize how differences in context, often patterned by race/ethnicity and socioeconomic status, came to be (Resnicow and Page 2008; Sanders Thompson 2009). Therefore, it is helpful to consider the use of theories that intentionally consider sociohistorical factors and incorporate these factors into the shaping of context and subsequent health behaviors and health inequities. Next, I discuss two theories, critical race theory and fundamental cause theory, that center equity and can be used by researchers and practitioners. These are by no means the only two theories that could be applied, but rather, these are highlighted as an example of a non–health- and a health-related example of how theories can be used to advance health equity goals.

Critical Race Theory

Critical race theory (CRT) emphasizes how pervasive and impactful racism is and provides a theoretical framework to connect racism to a wide variety of health outcomes (Ford and Airhihenbuwa 2018; Thomas et al. 2011).

Ford and Airhihenbuwa (2010, p. S32) define CRT as "an iterative methodology for helping investigators remain attentive to equity while carrying out research, scholarship, and practice. [CRT] urges scholars to work to transform the hierarchies they identify through research; draws on theory, experiential knowledge, and critical consciousness to illuminate and combat root causes of structural racism." CRT emphasizes the "permanence of race" by imploring researchers and practitioners to examine how racism has shaped social, historical, and contextual roots that fuel contemporary health inequities (Ford and Airhihenbuwa 2010; Gilbert and Ray 2016). For example, one key CRT concept is critical race consciousness, which advises scholars and practitioners to understand the key historical underpinnings of health inequities. Critical race consciousness encourages scholars to consider the long-lasting legacy of racism that has structured the inequitable distribution of resources and opportunities and driven observed inequities in various outcomes such as socioeconomics and health. CRT theorists argue that analyses of health inequities that do not accurately account for the role of racism reinforce the same structures that created inequities in the first place (Bonilla-Silva 2014; Bonilla-Silva and Baiocchi 2001; Ford and Airhihenbuwa 2010). For example, following the Great Depression, the US implemented the New Deal, including policies like the Social Security Act, US Housing Authority loans, and the GI Bill (Katznelson 2005; Rothstein 2017), which were designed to offer socioeconomic help to Americans. These policies were not equitably implemented, intentionally excluding Black Americans and other people of color from the transformational benefits that White people enjoyed. The inequitable distribution of New Deal–era policies, along with practices such as redlining, exacerbated inequities in housing, schools, infrastructure, and other key resources that have persisted into contemporary times (Thorpe et al. 2015). Considering how pivotal context is in relation to health, especially as it relates to health-promoting resources and services, any path to racial health equity must include disruptions to widespread racial residential segregation (Thorpe et al. 2015; Williams and Collins 2001).

Another aspect of CRT is to privilege the voices of those who have experiential knowledge of being marginalized in order to highlight where interventions should be directed (Ford and Airhihenbuwa 2010). "Centering at the margins" moves the lived experience of people, including scholars, from various marginalized backgrounds to the center (Ford and Airhihenbuwa 2010; Morse et al. 2020). As described above, community engagement is a proven approach to privileging historically marginalized voices (Goodman and Sanders Thompson 2017; Israel et al. 2018). Authentic community engagement often yields more effective, relevant strategies and solutions to health inequities because they incorporate the perspectives of community members, who are experts in their own lived experiences (Goodman et al. 2017). Incorporating the use of storytelling and narrative is an effective way to highlight the lived experience of community members and speak truth to power and advocate for shifts in power dynamics in order to center equity (Petteway 2019; Tsui and Starecheski 2018). Public health scholars have developed the Public Health Critical Race Praxis as a theoretical approach to connecting CRT principles to health equity (Ford and Airhihenbuwa 2010; Gilbert and Ray 2016).

Fundamental Cause Theory

Fundamental cause theory (FCT) is another theoretical approach that centers equity and helps researchers and practitioners to identify where power is located. One of the main premises of FCT is that power and social conditions such as racism and socioeconomic factors are fundamental in the patterning of health and well-being (Link and Phelan 1995). Fundamental social causes include access to resources, such as money, power, prestige, and access to the most desirable neighborhoods, which protect health and limit exposures that are deleterious to health across multiple outcomes (Link et al. 2008; Link and Phelan 1995). Therefore, FCT is an appropriate theory to guide researchers and practitioners who are interested in disrupting deeply entrenched power dynamics and to make strides toward equity. There are three main tenets of FCT: (1) individual-level risk factors must be contextualized to fully understand how broader factors affect levels of risk; (2) resources can be used to avoid risks and minimize the effects of exposures; and (3) fundamental causes affect multiple disease pathways and outcomes and continue to affect disease outcomes even when risk profiles change (Link and Phelan 1995). Juxtaposed against individual health behavior theories, FCT theorists argue that any efforts to address population-level factors by intervening at the individual level will fall flat. In their seminal paper, Link and Phelan argue that if fundamental causes are not addressed, marginalized populations will remain most at risk, no matter what the disease or health condition may be (Link and Phelan 1995).

FCT centers equity by focusing on upstream determinants of health, including power and the recognition that population-level health inequities require population-level solutions (Link et al. 2008; Link and Phelan, 1995). This calls for thinking beyond individual risk factors to consider not only how context shapes health behavior but how the social and physical environment are embodied within individuals' bodies (Krieger 2001; Rose 2001) and how that context needs to be changed to maximize the potential for individual shifts in behavior. For example, if individuals live in resource-constrained, stressful environments, they consistently experience unresolvable stressors that accumulate across the life course. Chronic stress is especially pernicious to health, and without considering ways to disrupt the structural inequities, disproportionate burdens of stress will continue to drive health inequities (Geronimus et al. 2006; 2016; Hicken et al. 2018). Simultaneously, the environment limits health-promoting resources and positive health behaviors such as safe places to recreate. Some scholars have found that people may use coping resources that are readily accessible and socially acceptable in their environments, such as consuming "comfort foods," but that while effective in helping to cope with stress in the short-term, are deleterious to health in the long-term (Jackson et al. 2010; Mezuk et al. 2011). FCT theorists encourage researchers and practitioners to adopt an "upstream" approach to solving health inequities by emphasizing factors that impact the population level, stretching beyond individual health behaviors (Williams et al. 2008).

Nonetheless, large-scale, radical structural changes are difficult to develop and implement (Rose 2001). Notwithstanding the formidable fiscal costs and political opposition, it is difficult to demonstrate the effectiveness of population-level solutions. Even if solutions are not at the population level, FCT theorists recommend that individual risk factors and health behaviors be contextualized, understanding the social, economic, and environmental forces that influence individual-level health behaviors (Link and Phelan 1995). This is an important theoretical perspective to maintain when developing solutions that primarily target individual behaviors, such as health behavior interventions. Furthermore, the FCT theoretical perspective is helpful to delineate where spheres of influence are and where to advocate for additional resources. For example, if a planning group is interested in improving physical activity, FCT may help the group to understand the feasibility of their intervention approach. It may also serve as a catalyst to advocate for specific resources such as the installation of bicycle lanes, development of culturally appropriate physical activity options, and the creation of green spaces.

Dissemination and Implementation Considerations

The field of dissemination and implementation has rapidly grown over the last decade as more and more scholars enter the field seeking ways to accelerate the development of evidence-based practices and the full-scale implementation of these best practices (Aarons et al. 2011, 2012; Proctor et al. 2009; Proctor and Brownson 2012). It is important to consider how to center equity in these processes as well.

When determining how to optimally implement a best practice, it is important to determine the barriers that impede implementation. Through an equity lens, it is important to ensure that there are adequate resources, including personnel and funding, to implement an evidence-based practice. Inequities in resources pose a major threat to firmly establishing whether best practices are relevant and effective in different contexts. If the costs of implementation are too high, individuals, agencies, and organizations will simply not invest in the implementation of an approach.

The cumulative management of research teams dedicated to health equity is critical to developing the evidence needed to motivate change and strive toward equity. The academic literature is replete with guidance about how to manage academic-community partnerships (Goodman and Sanders Thompson 2017; Hudson et al. 2023; Israel et al. 2018). However, there is less information about how to manage a research team with an equity lens. For example, health equity researchers may find that their staff resides in the same areas as their research participants, faced with the same social, economic, and environmental challenges. For example, some research staff may feel self-conscious as they ask participants about financial security or housing challenges when they are experiencing the same stressors. Similarly, when there is harm within the broader community, it is likely that this is affecting research staff as well. While accounting for the lived experiences of research staff may enhance the research being conducted, it is a delicate balance to avoid making staff feel embarrassed or tokenized. For example, in the aftermath of public, police-involved killings of unarmed Black men in places like Minneapolis and St. Louis, researchers have found that Black people in predominantly White spaces were often compelled to explain complex, decades-long inequities and the subsequent frustration, anger, and heartbreak of communities that were long oppressed while still processing their own feelings (Hudson 2021; Hudson et al. 2016). Additionally, some Black Americans may not feel that their perspectives are representative of all Black Americans or that they may not even know enough to characterize certain events. These are factors that are likely occurring on research teams throughout the country as individual researchers, community partners, staffers, and even students are simultaneously coping with their own everyday stressors, which are often related to the same topics that are being studied, while also maintaining professionalism and doing their jobs to the best of their ability. These are factors that are likely to affect the implementation of projects and compel researchers and practitioners to consider how to better center equity in the research process.

Another challenge in implementation is how to best disseminate knowledge and processes, especially to individuals and communities that have been historically marginalized and may not have adequate resources to invest in the adoption of a best practice (Aarons et al. 2012). Academic-based researchers and practitioners must consider whether their research findings are accessible to the communities they seek to serve. Many community-based practitioners and private citizens do not have access to academic journals, and the cost of this access is beyond the capacity of most. It is critical to think about dissemination on the front end and work with community-based partners to figure out what the most effective, accessible ways to share information might be. In addition to peer-reviewed publishing, it may be appropriate to distribute newsletters that describe the progress of the research team. Face-to-face meetings such as gatherings over meals or during resource fairs can also be helpful and make it easier for community partners and research participants to learn more about the research that is occurring. This also encourages reciprocity, such that researchers are providing information and resources to communities rather than just extracting data. Hosting public forums is another way to gather feedback about the approach to research and the interpretation of study findings. For example, community cafes have been shown to be an effective way to engage people from different disciplines and experiences in dialogue, with the goal of developing solutions to a broad range of inequities. No matter what the channel and specific approach may be, it is critical to plan for dissemination from the start. This will allow researchers, practitioners, and community partners to consider how to make an equitable dissemination plan.

Many resources are widely available to aid in the dissemination of findings to different audiences. For researchers and practitioners interested in policy development and advocacy, there are trainings to help translate findings and develop relationships with policy-makers at different levels. For example, among academic-based researchers, there is the Scholars Strategy Network, which helps to connect researchers to key stakeholders (e.g., elected officials and journalists) to motivate change. Academy Health offers regular webinars and other virtual training opportunities in addition to their annual research meeting and dissemination and implementation conference.

Conclusion

Centering equity in research requires the intentional consideration of equity throughout the entire research process, from ideation to dissemination. It is critical to engage, authentically, with community members to develop the most appropriate lens to characterize health inequities and to craft the most effective solutions to inequities. Authentic community engagement is often a long process, so there is a need to improve the value of this work within academic spaces and other research settings to make sure the process of community engagement is not undermined by pressure to align research aims and questions with the funding priorities of different agencies and foundations. Rather, it is critical to center efforts and investments on the needs community members identify and find to be the most relevant.

Theory is often underutilized in general among public health researchers and practitioners, which makes it more difficult to identify and disseminate best practices. For scholars and practitioners dedicated to health equity, it is even more imperative to develop and use theories that accurately capture the complex sociohistorical factors that drive contemporary health inequities across race/ethnicity, gender, socioeconomic status, and other status-, power-, and identity-related characteristics. The theories highlighted in this chapter, CRT and FCT, also provide a lens to examine power and, based on that analysis, where the most appropriate levers of intervention may be.

Equity must be centered in the implementation and dissemination process. While a thorough discussion of centering equity in research methods, analysis, and interpretation of results is beyond the scope of this chapter, there are key considerations to bear in mind throughout the research process, particularly for scholars and practitioners interested in the development of interventions. The selection of an appropriate theoretical framework that centers equity will provide a scaffolding to guide the development of interventions. During the implementation process, it is important to share study methods, processes, and findings broadly, creating avenues to disseminate in an equitable manner. Maintaining a diverse research team that is representative of the population in which the research is being conducted can add value to the quality of inquiry. However, there is a balance necessary to be sensitive to staff that may be residing in and living through the same stressors and contexts as the research catchment area. Similarly, it may be important to consider how power and privilege are showing up on research teams and within community partnerships.

There is no prescriptive, ultimate guide to centering equity in research. However, the scholarship in this area is continuing to grow, and the evidence is seen in the development of new funding initiatives, the formation of new research questions, and meetings that allow people to share what they have learned. Because this area is still growing and is organic in so many ways, there is no substitute for experience. Nonetheless, embracing humility and curiosity will aid in the development of fruitful partnerships where norms of mutual respect are observed. These partnerships help research teams center equity, and where conflict arises, remembering the common goals and mutual intentions among team members and revisiting a shared theoretical framework helps to keep research on track.

References

Aarons, G. A., G. Cafri, L. Lugo, and A. Sawitzky. 2012. "Expanding the Domains of Attitudes towards Evidence-Based Practice: The Evidence Based Attitudes Scale-50." *Administration and Policy in Mental Health and Mental Health Services Research* (5): 331–340.

Aarons, G. A., M. Hurlburt, and S. M. Horwitz. 2011. "Advancing a Conceptual Model of Evidence-Based Practice Implementation in Public Service Sectors." *Adm Policy Ment Health* 38: 4–23.

Bonilla-Silva, Eduardo. 2014. *Racism without Racists: Color-Blind Racism and the Persistence of Racial Inequality in America.* New York, Rowman and Littlefield.

Bonilla-Silva, Eduardo, and Gianpaolo Baiocchi. 2001. "Anything but Racism: How Sociologists Limit the Significance of Racism." *Race and Society* 4 (2): 117–131.

Braveman, Paula. 2006. "Health Disparities and Health Equity: Concepts and Measurement." *Annual Review of Public Health* 27: 167–194.

Braveman, Paula, Susan Egerter, and David R. Williams. 2011. "The Social Determinants of Health: Coming of Age." *Annual Review of Public Health* 32: 381–398.

Carpiano, Richard M., and Dorothy M. Daley. 2006. "A Guide and Glossary on Postpositivist Theory Building for Population Health." *Journal of Epidemiology and Community Health* 60 (7): 564–570.

Ford, Chandra L., and Collins O. Airhihenbuwa. 2010. "Critical Race Theory, Race Equity, and Public Health: Toward Antiracism Praxis." *American Journal of Public Health* 100 (Suppl 1): S30–S35.

Ford, Chandra L., and Collins O. Airhihenbuwa. 2018. "Commentary: Just What Is Critical Race Theory and What's It Doing in a Progressive Field like Public Health?" *Ethnicity & Disease* 28 (Suppl 1): 223–230.

Freire, Kimberley E., Leah Perkinson, Susan Morrel-Samuels, and Marc A. Zimmerman. 2015. "Three Cs of Translating Evidence-Based Programs for Youth and Families to Practice Settings." *New Directions for Child and Adolescent Development* 2015 (149): 25–39.

Geronimus, Arline T., Cynthia. G. Colen, Tara Shochet, L. B. Ingber, and Sherman A. James. 2006. "Urban-Rural Differences in Excess Mortality among High-Poverty Populations: Evidence from the Harlem Household Survey and the Pitt County, North Carolina Study of African American Health." *Journal of Health Care for the Poor and Underserved* 17 (3): 532–558.

Geronimus, Arline T., Sherman A. James, Mesmin Destin, Louis A. Graham, Mark Hatzenbuehler, Mary Murphy, Jay A. Pearson, Amel Omari, and James Phillip Thompson. 2016. "Jedi Public Health: Co-Creating an Identity-Safe Culture to Promote Health Equity." *SSM - Population Health* 2 (March): 105–116.

Gilbert, Keon L., and Rashawn Ray. 2016. "Why Police Kill Black Males with Impunity: Applying Public Health Critical Race Praxis (PHCRP) to Address the Determinants of Policing Behaviors and 'Justifiable' Homicides in the USA." *Journal of Urban Health: Bulletin of the New York Academy of Medicine* 93 (Suppl 1): 122–140.

Gollust, Sarah E., Kathleen T. Call, J. Robin Moon, Bonnie Cluxton, and Zinzi Bailey. 2022. "Designing and Implementing a Curriculum to Support Health Equity Research Leaders: The Interdisciplinary Research Leaders Experience." *Frontiers in Public Health* 10: 876847.

Goodman, Melody S., and Vetta L. Sanders Thompson. 2017. "The Science of Stakeholder Engagement in Research: Classification, Implementation, and Evaluation." *Translational Behavioral Medicine* 7 (3): 486–491.

Goodman, Melody S., and Vetta L. Sanders Thompson. 2018. *Public Health Research Methods for Partnerships and Practice.* New York: Routledge.

Hicken, Margaret T., Nicole Kravitz-Wirtz, Myles Durkee, and James S. Jackson. 2018. "Racial Inequalities in Health: Framing Future Research." *Social Science & Medicine* 199: 11–18.

Hudson, Darrell. 2021. "Achieving Health Equity by Addressing Legacies of Racial Violence in Public Health Practice." *Annals of the American Academy of Political and Social Science* 694 (1): 59–66.

Hudson, Darrell. 2023. "Developing Antiracist Research to Address Racial/Ethnic Health and Socioeconomic Inequities: Conceptual Frameworks that Guide Equity." *Journal of the Society for Social Work and Research* 14 (1): 151–163.

Hudson, Darrell, Keon Gilbert, and Melody Goodman. 2023. "Promoting Authentic Academic-Community Engagement to Advance Health Equity." *International Journal of Environmental Research and Public Health* 20 (4): 2874.

Hudson, Darrell L., Jake Eaton, Andrae Banks, Whitney Sewell, and Harold Neighbors. 2016. "'Down in the Sewers': Perceptions of Depression and Depression Care among African American Men." *American Journal of Men's Health* 12 (1): 126–137.

Israel, Barbara A., A. J. Schulz, E. A. Parker, A. B. Becker, A. J. Allen, R. Guzman, and Richard Lichtenstein. 2018. "Critical Issues in Developing and Following CBPR Principles." In *Community-Based Participatory Research for Health: Advancing Social and Health Equity*, edited by N. Wallenstein, Bonnie Duran, J. G. Gotzel, and M. Minkler, 31–47. New Jersey: Jossey-Bass Hoboken.

Jackson, James S., Katherine M. Knight, and Jane A. Rafferty. 2010. "Race and Unhealthy Behaviors: Chronic Stress, the HPA Axis, and Physical and Mental Health Disparities over the Life Course." *American Journal of Public Health* 100 (5): 933–939.

Jagosh, Justin, Ann C. Macaulay, Pierre Pluye, Jon Salsberg, Paula L. Bush, Jim Henderson, Erin Sirett, et al. 2012. "Uncovering the Benefits of Participatory Research: Implications of a Realist Review for Health Research and Practice." *Milbank Quarterly* 90 (2): 311–46.

Katznelson, I. 2005. *When Affirmative Action Was White: An Untold Story of Racial Inequality in Twentieth Century America*. New York: W.W. Norton & Co.

Komaie, Goldie, Christine C. Ekenga, Vetta L. Sanders Thompson, and Melody S. Goodman. 2017. "Increasing Community Research Capacity to Address Health Disparities." *Journal of Empirical Research on Human Research Ethics* 12 (1): 55–66.

Krieger, N. 2001. "Theories for Social Epidemiology in the 21st Century: An Ecosocial Perspective." *International Journal of Epidemiology* 30: 668–677.

Link, B. G., and J. C. Phelan. 1995. "Social Conditions as Fundamental Causes of Disease." *Journal of Health and Social Behavior* Extra Issue: 80–94. PMID: 7560851.

Link, Bruce G., Jo C. Phelan, Richard Miech, and Emily Leckman Westin. 2008. "The Resources that Matter: Fundamental Social Causes of Health Disparities and the Challenge of Intelligence." *Journal of Health and Social Behavior* 49 (1): 72–91.

Martinez, Jenny, Carin Wong, Catherine Verrier Piersol, Dawn Clayton Bieber, Bonita L. Perry, and Natalie E. Leland. 2019. "Stakeholder Engagement in Research: A Scoping Review of Current Evaluation Methods." *Journal of Comparative Effectiveness Research* 8 (15): 1327–1341.

Mattessich, P. W., and K. M. Johnson. 2018. *Collaboration: What Makes It Work*. Nashville, Tn: Fieldstone Alliance.

Mezuk, Briana, Jane A. Rafferty, Kiarri N. Kershaw, Darrell Hudson, Cleopatra M. Abdou, Hedwig Lee, William W. Eaton, and James S. Jackson. 2011. "Reconsidering the Role of Social Disadvantage in Physical and Mental Health: Stressful Life

Events, Health Behaviors, Race, and Depression." *American Journal of Epidemiology* 172 (11): 1238–1239.

Morrel-Samuels, Susan, Martica Bacallao, Shelli Brown, Meredith Bower, and Marc Zimmerman. 2016. "Community Engagement in Youth Violence Prevention: Crafting Methods to Context." *Journal of Primary Prevention* 37 (2): 189–207.

Morse, Michelle, Amy Finnegan, Bram Wispelwey, and Chandra Ford. 2020. Will COVID-19 Pave the Way for Progressive Social Policies? Insights from Critical Race Theory. Health Affairs, July 2, https://doi.org/10.1377/forefront.20200630.18403.

Petteway, Ryan J. 2019. "Intergenerational Photovoice Perspectives of Place and Health in Public Housing: Participatory Coding, Theming, and Mapping in/of the 'Structure Struggle.'" *Health & Place* 60: 102229.

Proctor, E. K., and R. C. Brownson. 2012. "Measurement Issues in Dissemination and Implementation Research." Edited by R. C. Brownson, G. A. Colditz, and E. K. Proctor. New York: Oxford University Press.

Proctor, E. K., J. Landsverk, G. Aarons, D. Chambers, C. Glisson, and B. Mittman. 2009. "Implementation Research in Mental Health Services: An Emerging Science with Conceptual, Methodological, and Training Challenges." *Administration and Policy in Mental Health and Mental Health Services Research* 36 (1): 24–34.

Resnicow, Kenneth, and Scott E. Page. 2008. "Embracing Chaos and Complexity: A Quantum Change for Public Health." *American Journal of Public Health* 98 (8): 1382–1389.

Rose, G. 2001. "Sick Individuals and Sick Populations." *International Journal of Epidemiology* 30 (3): 427–432.

Rothstein, Richard. 2017. *The Color of Law: A Forgotten History of How Our Government Segregated America.* New York: W.W. Norton & Co.

Sanders Thompson, Vetta L. 2009. "Cultural Context and Modification of Behavior Change Theory." *Health Education & Behavior* 36 (Suppl 5suppl): 156S–160S.

Syme, S. L. 2008. "Reducing Racial and Social-Class Inequalities in Health: The Need for a New Approach." *Health Affairs* 27 (2): 456–459.

Syme, S. Leonard. 2005. "Historical Perspective: The Social Determinants of Disease – Some Roots of the Movement." *Epidemiologic Perspectives & Innovations* 2 (1): 2.

Thomas, Stephen B., Sandra Crouse Quinn, James Butler, Craig S. Fryer, and Mary A. Garza. 2011. "Toward a Fourth Generation of Disparities Research to Achieve Health Equity." *Annual Review of Public Health* 32: 399–416.

Thorpe, Roland J., Elizabeth Kelley, Janice V. Bowie, Derek M. Griffith, Marino Bruce, and Thomas LaVeist. 2015. "Explaining Racial Disparities in Obesity among Men: Does Place Matter?" *American Journal of Men's Health* 9 (6): 464–472.

Tsui, E. K., and A. Starecheski. 2018. "Uses of Oral History and Digital Storytelling in Public Health Research and Practice." *Public Health* 154 (January): 24–30.

Whitehead, Margaret, Bo Burström, and Finn Diderichsen. 2000. "Social Policies and the Pathways to Inequalities in Health: A Comparative Analysis of Lone Mothers in Britain and Sweden." *Social Science & Medicine* 50 (2): 255–270.

Williams, David R., and Chiquita Collins. 2001. "Racial Residential Segregation: A Fundamental Cause of Racial Disparities in Health." *Public Health Reports* 116 (5): 404–416.

Williams, David R., Manuela V. Costa, Adebola O. Odunlami, and Selina A. Mohammed. 2008. "Moving Upstream: How Interventions that Address the Social Determinants of Health Can Improve Health and Reduce Disparities." *Journal of Public Health Management and Practice* 14 (6): S8–S17.

Chapter 6
Privilege and Intersectionality Frameworks in Public Health

Greta Bauer

Privilege and Marginalization

In understanding health, we accept that social power, privilege, and oppression are not abstract social constructs. They shape the frequency and severity of health-harming experiences, the frequency and extremity of health-enhancing experiences, and the opportunities that are open or foreclosed for people as they navigate their lives. These experiences are not distributed equally across a population, and their patterning also plays a role in shaping an individual person's expectations about what is likely—or even possible—for people like them. Moreover, some experiences may directly change one's embodiment, as social experiences become inscribed into anatomy and physiology through disease or injury, ideal or nonideal healing, tooth decay, cortisol levels, or up- or downregulation of cellular production of specific proteins. Again, these effects will not be distributed equally across populations.

How then are those of us with a commitment to health equity to understand the ways that social power, privilege, and marginalization shape experiences for different groups within a population? Health research has increasingly addressed stigma and discrimination, particularly the types that are enacted in interpersonal interactions (Stuber et al. 2008). Does this provide a theoretical framework to inform the broader picture we need to understand health equity and health itself? Absolutely. Could we take this further? Again, yes. Incorporating the additional frameworks of social privilege and intersectionality has the potential to create a richer understanding.

Greta Bauer, *Privilege and Intersectionality Frameworks in Public Health*. In: *Power, Privilege, and Public Health in the United States*. Edited by: Lorraine T. Dean and Keilah A. Jacques, Oxford University Press. © Oxford University Press (2025). DOI: 10.1093/9780197760956.003.0006

Conceptualizing Privilege: Not Simply a Lack of Discrimination

Conceptualizations of privilege draw heavily on Peggy McIntosh's formative work on White privilege from the late 1980s, which can be extended or adapted to other types of privilege. McIntosh conceptualizes White privilege as an invisible and weightless backpack of tools that White people carry with them, including "special provisions, maps, passports, codebooks, visas, clothes, tools, and blank checks" (McIntosh 2019). While privilege is more than a lack of experience of discrimination, some of these privileges do represent this absence, and McIntosh characterizes these as within the first of two types of experiences of privilege. Examples include not being followed or harassed when shopping alone, not being dropped from a list of job finalists for having an appropriate but foreign education, and being able to go out dressed sloppily without anyone attributing the sloppiness to the character of members of your group. She describes these types of experiences as what we would wish for everyone in a just world. We can call these types of privileged experiences *just and fair experience*. In addition to nondiscrimination, just and fair experiences include those related to integration within society, such as ease of finding a hairdresser with experience cutting hair like one's own. Just and fair experiences are those that should be experienced by everyone in a just and fair society. There is nothing wrong or harmful about experiencing them, but the privilege is in both the experience and the expectation of fair treatment.

Other experiences of privilege, however, constitute a license for ignorance, and McIntosh argues that, unlike just and fair experiences, these types of privilege create harm for both the one holding the privilege and those subjected to that ignorance (McIntosh 2019). An example would be holding the unchallenged belief that White Europeans built civilization, ignoring the many advanced civilizations built by Black and Brown nations throughout Africa, Asia, Australia, and the Americas. We can call these privileged experiences *allowed harmful ignorance*. Allowed harmful ignorance extends to beliefs about other individuals and groups, as well as one's own.

As a result of this distinction between these two types of privilege, in 1989 McIntosh called for a "more finely differentiated taxonomy of privilege" (McIntosh 2019). Since then, not a lot of progress has been made toward an explicit and expanded taxonomy. However, McIntosh's conceptualization of white privilege as tools that either grant what all should have or allow ignorance can be adapted for application to different privileged groups and expanded to more than two dimensions of privilege. In Figure 6.1, I build on

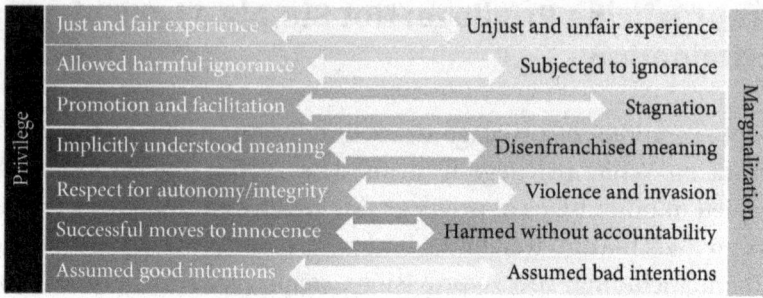

Figure 6.1 Sevenfold gradient of individual experiences of privilege and marginalization.
Source: Conceptualized and designed by the author. Licensed by Greta Bauer under CC BY 4.0. To view a copy of this license, visit https://creativecommons.org/licenses/by/4.0/.

McIntosh's two dimensions of White privilege to develop a sevenfold gradient of privilege that applies to not only White privilege but to privilege associated with ability, sexual orientation, gender, ethnic, or religious group, or other social categories across which social power is structured. With experiences of social marginalization positioned as the other pole, McIntosh's two initial dimensions are reflected by their converses: unjust and unfair experience and being subjected to ignorance about those like you.

The first of the five added dimensions of privilege are those that actively facilitate positive experiences or advance one's life. If discrimination and its counterpart in daily microaggressions create barriers and friction in one's movement through the world, there are also processes that not only lower barriers but lubricate interpersonal interactions and social inclusion and advancement (Bauer 2014). The absence of discrimination in a job setting might be a privilege, but it is not the same privilege as someone tapping you on the shoulder to say "Hey, I think you would be a good fit for this leadership role," for example. This experience is more likely to happen for those who match an implicitly understood profile of what a leader looks like. We can label this third type of privilege *promotion and facilitation*. It happens when others open up opportunities and lubricate your movement forward in life or when this is created structurally—for example through legacy admissions to prestigious universities based on parental attendance. When this force that moves lives along a positive trajectory is not present, stagnation may result relative to others with similar skills, abilities, and resources.

We can add yet another category when we consider shared meanings that make one's experience intelligible and communicable. If, for example, your cultural understanding does not differentiate between sexual orientation and gender identity, but melds these together within social and ceremonial gendered roles as in some Indigenous communities (Canadian Institutes of Health Research, Institute of Gender and Health et al. 2020; Jacobs et al. 1997), it will take more effort to communicate this understanding than it would to communicate a "mainstream" public health understanding or sexual orientation and gender identity as two distinct concepts. The privilege of *implicitly understood meaning* allows people to see representations of themselves, answer survey questions while fitting into a listed response option, refer to their holidays by name without definition, and not have the burden of communicating (or being too exhausted to communicate) many aspects of the specifics of one's race, ethnicity and culture, disability, religion, sexuality, or gender. While some burden of explanation is expected in communication and is unavoidable, the repeated nature of this work places a differential burden on some members of society. It may also disadvantage in other ways— for example, when needing to provide more background explanation in a word-limited scholarship essay, leaving less space for key content.

Violence, coercion, and physically invasive experiences stand in their own category, distinct from discrimination. Oppression can be enacted through physical or sexual violence, or the threat of violence, and through coercion and control. Patricia Hill Collins writes that social patterns of violence can tell us a lot about how power is structured within a society because, simply put, "people don't go willingly to their assigned places" (Collins 2019). In contrast, privilege can be understood as *respect for autonomy and bodily integrity*. This includes protection from violence and coercive control of one's body, movement, and actions. It includes the ability to make medical decisions without spousal consent and not to be restricted from living or being present in a geographic area based on one's group membership. It also includes experiencing daily acts of respect, such as having others respect your space and not touch your hair, pregnant belly, or other body parts without permission.

Moves to innocence are acts of privilege that attempt to deny or obscure one's role in perpetuating oppression (Mawhinney 1998). Tuck and Yang (Tuck and Yang, 2012) identify types of moves to innocence in the context of decolonization, including claims of nebulous Indigenous ancestry that serve to deflect blame, settler adoption fantasies (or "going native"), creating ambiguity between actual decolonization of land and general anti-imperialist struggles, focusing solely on decolonizing the mind, representing Indigenous people in data as either "at risk" or invisibilized as uncounted or footnoted, and settler reoccupation and urban homesteading. Outside of a decolonization framework, moves to innocence may similarly involve nebulous claims of in-group membership or proximity (e.g., "but some of my best friends are. . ."), stated allyship without corresponding action, shifting focus onto similarity of individual experiences to deflect from structural causes of oppression, declarations of color blindness or failure to see other differences, and ongoing erasure of marginalized groups from data or policies. Moves to innocence support the retention of privilege through concealing any complicity in oppression and through relief of guilt and responsibility (Tuck and Yang 2012).

Finally, *assumed good intentions* can produce the privilege of nonaccountability for harmful words or actions, including acts that marginalize others though the other mechanisms (Figure 6.1). The assumption of good intentions may produce social pressure for those who recognize oppressive harms to acknowledge the nonintentional nature of oppression and to expend energy relieving actors of guilt or blame.

By identifying these seven dimensions of privilege, we can see that experiences along the privilege-to-marginalization gradient may be marked by differences in discrimination, violence, ignorance, meaning, and promotion, with harm to others excused through both moves to innocence and assumptions of good intentions. A full experience of privilege may be hard to discern for those experiencing it. Respect for bodily integrity, fair experiences, and appropriate promotion and facilitation should be the norm, so awareness of these types of privilege emerges only with the recognition that others are not being treated similarly. Implicitly understood meaning, allowing of ignorance, and assumption of good intentions are typically privileges extended to majority groups and, as such, may be experienced by those without consistent challenge from individuals or information outside these groups. Even in cases where numeric minority groups may be culturally and politically dominant, a deep history of dominance embeds itself in culture and language, including education, civic holidays, street names, and policies, in such a way as to make dominant cultural references near-universally understood.

Multiple Privileges, Multiple Marginalizations

This idea of marginalization and privilege or power as poles on a spectrum is most typically understood as unidimensional, showcasing White privilege, male privilege, heteronormativity, or other singular types of privilege. However, no one person's life is lived out in a single dimension, and few people's lives are positioned at exclusively privileged or exclusively marginalized positions. How then should we think about multiple privileges or privileges in the context of other marginalizations?

Gradients of privilege to marginalization are often mapped onto multiple social categories—for example, through wheel models. Many versions and adaptations of such wheels of power and privilege exist. The wheel in Figure 6.2 is from a "Meet the Methods" document produced to highlight my work by the Canadian Institutes for Health Research's (CIHR's) Institute of Gender and Health (Canadian Institutes of Health Research, Institute of Gender and Health and Bauer 2021). It is adapted from artist Sylvia Duckworth's wheel, which in turn combines others, citing specifically a Canadian Council for Refugees' version of the wheel. These types of models are often customized; thus, this Canadian wheel privileges English and French languages and visually highlights the sex and gender wedges.

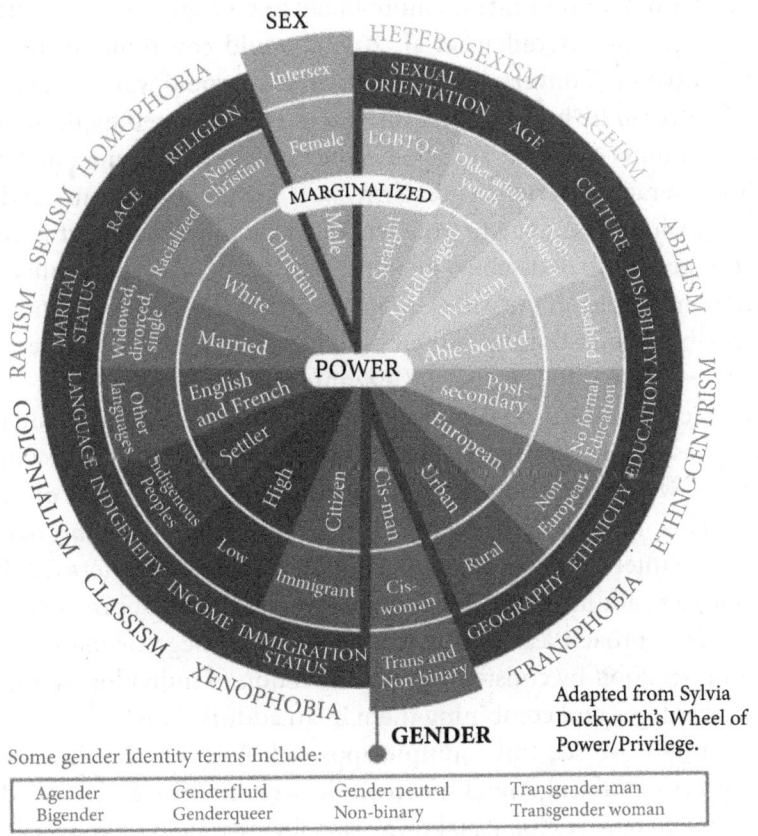

Some gender Identity terms Include:

| Agender | Genderfluid | Gender neutral | Transgender man |
| Bigender | Genderqueer | Non-binary | Transgender woman |

Adapted from Sylvia Duckworth's Wheel of Power/Privilege.

Figure 6.2 Wheel of Power and Privilege from the Institute of Gender and Health at the Canadian Institutes of Health Research.
Source: Sex-gender-power-wheel © 2021 by CIHR, adapted from Sylvia Duckworth. Wheel of Power/Privilege is licensed under CC BY 4.0. To view a copy of this license, visit http://creativecommons.org/licenses/by/4.0/.
Note: This figure is available in full color online at Oxford Academic.

Such wheel models show privilege as centered and marginalization as literally at the margins of the wheel. The processes giving rise to this (e.g., racism) are explicitly labeled around the perimeter. Thus, it is possible to see how, for example, Black women could be marginalized within both antiracism and feminist/antisexist projects; this marginalization was the basis for Crenshaw's metaphor of intersectionality (Bello 2016).

Each wedge represents the gradient from a privileged center to a marginalized periphery and can thus be mapped onto the sevenfold gradient of privilege and marginalization. We can easily produce examples of how this might play out through experience. For example, the race wedge shows White people as privileged and racialized people as more marginalized. Racial discrimination in hiring, more likely to be experienced by Black and Latino/a/x persons (Quillian et al. 2017), would constitute an unjust and unfair experience. Conversely, the experience we would want for everyone— fair evaluation in hiring—is more likely to be experienced by those who are White. As another example, able-bodied persons, near the center of the wheel, would on average experience greater respect for their autonomy and bodily integrity during pregnancy (a time where a lack of such respect is common across categories) than disabled persons. Those with visible mobility disabilities, more marginal on the wheel, report both invasive touching and invasive or disgust-based questioning of their bodies, as well as repeated interrogation of processes that led to pregnancy (Iezzoni et al. 2015).

Thus, such wheel models combine well with the sevenfold gradient if we imagine these gradients to apply in a universal way where privilege within one of a wheel's wedges is independent of one's positioning on each of the other wedges. This represents a *multiple-privilege or multiple-marginalization approach*. In intersectionality scholarship, this is sometimes termed the multiple approach, additive approach, or non-intersectional approach (Hancock 2007). This approach assumes that a person's privilege or marginalization may be understood by considering the collection of individual marginalizations or privileges and combining them in an additive way.

Where might we see this multiple approach in public health and equity work? Diversity training sometimes includes a common exercise called a privilege walk, where participants take one step forward, remain in place, or take one step backward in response to a series of questions about specific indicators of privilege or marginalization, such as parents' education, comfort with disclosing sexual orientation, or safety of their neighborhoods. At the end of the exercise, participants look around to see their position relative to those of their peers, having created a visual privilege-to-marginalization gradient with their bodies. While it might not be immediately intuitive, the main effects regression models used in public health research to statistically predict an outcome based on social status or position variables functionally mirror this same exercise. In statistical modeling, the "forward steps" or "backward steps" are of unequal size, as specified by the regression parameter estimates from the model. One might "step forward" for the average advantage value for males and "step backward" for the average disadvantage value for sexual minority persons, with each possible combination of social status or position categories producing an estimate for whatever the specified outcome is. Thus, as in the privilege walk, we can predict outcomes for each combination of categories or responses based on adding effects together.

Such multiple approaches are relatively common in health education and research. However, is there a reason to believe that this is how privilege and marginalization function—as effects that can just be added together? There is a wealth of public health examples to counter this assumption and to show that this type of additive relationship cannot be assumed. In qualitative research, it is clear that participants cannot clearly respond to questions asking them to disaggregate their experiences according to aspects of their social status (Bowleg 2008, 2013). In Bowleg's classic paper, this conclusion becomes part of the title: "Black + Lesbian + Woman ≠ Black Lesbian Woman" (Bowleg 2008). In quantitative research, examples and simulation studies show that this type of main effects regression will misestimate health outcomes for groups cross-coded from different social categories (e.g., Black men) (Bowleg and Bauer 2016; Mahendran et al. 2022a, 2022b), indicating that it is, in fact, not a good explanation for how privileges or marginalizations should be combined.

If we accept that the effects of one "type" of privilege or marginalization cannot be understood as independent of others, then the following situations could be true: (1) The degree of privilege or marginalization might vary depending on another social status. For example, postsecondary education (located near the power center of the wheel) might produce diminished returns among transgender and nonbinary people or any other group subject to high levels of employment discrimination, which may reduce the associated economic benefit. (2) What is viewed as "privileged" may be unclear or even reversed. For example, cisgender maleness (near the power center for both sex and gender) may generate risk rather than advantage for a young Black person with an intellectual disability in the context of anti-Black racism. As an exercise, we can consider the extent to which the following statement might be true for any combination: ___(category 1)___ may mitigate the [privilege/marginalization] of ___(category 2)___ in ___(context)___. For example, whiteness may mitigate the marginalization of being an immigrant in majority-White countries. Being LGBTQ+ may mitigate the privilege of being Christian in the United States. Thus, we can easily see that experiences of privilege and marginalization are interdependent.

Intersectionality

These examples of interdependence show the importance of incorporating an intersectional understanding of privilege and marginalization that can move us beyond ideas that privilege or marginalization operate independently across different axes of oppression, such as racism, sexism, or homophobia. In actuality, the original document containing the wheel in Figure 6.2 explicitly notes that "what constitutes a position of power may play out differently at different intersections and in different contexts" (Canadian Institutes of Health Research, Institute of Gender and Health and Bauer 2021). In other words, wheel models of power and privilege and other similar conceptualizations are not themselves intersectional.

Intersectionality theoretical frameworks emerged in public health only recently. A Black feminist theoretical framework, rooted in the complexity of social marginalization along race, class, gender, and sexual orientation (Combahee River Collective 1977) intersectionality has additional roots in Chicana and Native American feminisms (Collins and Bilge 2020, 72–100). Introduced into academic work through the work of Patricia Hill Collins in sociology (Collins, 1990) and Kimberlé Crenshaw in legal studies (Crenshaw 1989, 1991), intersectionality traveled rapidly across disciplines, sparking scholarship on its research applications by Ange-Marie Hancock in political science (Hancock 2007), Leslie McCall in sociology (McCall 2005), and Elizabeth Cole in psychology (Cole 2009). Only then did public health scholars begin to explicitly engage with how intersectionality could transform conceptualizations of difference in public health (Bowleg 2012) and approaches to population health research (Bauer 2014).

Intersectionality scholars take the approach that intersectionality is an "analytic sensibility" (Cho et al. 2013) and often present intersectional frameworks as thinking tools that we can use to apply to our areas of interest. The preceding section's discussion of how privilege functions has already introduced us to two of intersectionality's core ideas with high relevance to public health: oppression and relationality (Collins and Bilge 2020; Misra et al. 2021).

Oppression includes core intersectional ideas of social power, social inequality, and social justice (Collins and Bilge 2020, 72–100; Misra et al.

2021). Social power is the sine qua non of intersectionality (Bowleg and Bauer 2016; Collins 2015), and interlocking systems of power and oppression (Collins 1990) must underpin public health understandings of privilege and marginalization. Black feminist work explicitly concerns how social power shapes and constrains experiences across multiple axes of oppression in ways that are specific to intersectional social locations—the ways that race/ethnicity, sex/gender, social class, and sexual orientation are understood and treated in social context (Collins 1990; Combahee River Collective 1977; Davis 1983). It is this focus on interlocking systems of oppression that differentiates intersectional approaches to public health from sociodemographic analyses of health disparities or social determinants of health approaches.

The interdependence of experiences of privilege and marginalization discussed earlier also introduced us to the idea of *intersectional relationality*. Relationality helps us understand how privilege and marginalization cannot be understood along individual axes but only through how they are shaped by others (Collins 2019). One way to approach relationality is to ask what happens when we add a new category to one on which we might be focused (Collins 2019). What happens when we add gender into a focus on race, or sexism into a focus on racism? What happens when we add an understanding of socioeconomic status, race, sexual orientation, or gender to our focus on anti-immigrant discrimination? What happens when we add ability and disability, sexual orientation, family status, or stigmatized conditions or labels such as addiction, mental health diagnoses, or HIV-positive status? We can also ask how these previously separate privileges or marginalizations function differently when joined to each other. Finally, we can understand how sometimes this joining creates something new and co-formed that cannot be separated back into its components (Collins 2019).

Intersectional complexity, another of intersectionality's core ideas, is understood by scholars in different ways (Collins and Bilge 2020; McCall 2005; Misra et al. 2021). A useful distinction for those in public health is between intra-categorical and inter-categorical approaches to intersectional complexity (McCall 2005). Intra-categorical approaches explore or make visible the ways experience is shaped at specific social intersections in differing ways, while inter-categorical approaches focus on comparison across intersections.

Intra-categorical intersection-specific experiences are those that may be unique or have a unique character for those whose lives are lived out at a particular intersection. Even similar-seeming constructs may be shaped differently at different intersections. As an example, gendered racial microaggressions are the experiences of gendered racism (or racialized sexism) that represent relational formulations of day-to-day racism and sexism that play out to undermine equity. We can see how gendered racial microaggressions are formulated differently for different intersections by considering the results from two groups of researchers that set out to develop survey measures of gendered racial microaggressions. Both conducted mixed-method studies of US women, using qualitative data to develop their measure and quantitative data to validate it. Both produced survey measures with four subscales to measure different components of gendered racial microaggressions. That, however, is where the similarity ends, as the sets of subscales have no overlap. The Gendered Racial Microaggressions Scale for Asian American Women (GRMSAAW) included subscales of (1) ascription of submissiveness, (2) assumption of universal appearance, (3) Asian fetishism, and (4) media invalidation (Keum et al. 2018), while the Gendered Racial Microaggressions Scale (GRMS) for Black women produced subscales of (1) assumptions of beauty and sexual objectification, (2) silenced and marginalized, (3) strong black woman stereotype, and (4) angry black woman stereotype (Lewis and Neville 2015). The complete lack of overlap in subscales demonstrates how relational co-formation may produce processes of oppression that take distinct forms for those at different intersectional social locations. Such intersection-specific or intra-categorical constructs may be so distinct they cannot be meaningfully measured or compared across intersections.

Inter-categorical approaches focus on comparisons across intersections and have become increasingly used in public health research to take a more precise and community-relevant approach to health disparity research (Bauer et al. 2021; Bauer and Scheim 2019b; Evans et al. 2018; Guan et al. 2021). In the most common versions of such approaches, health disparities are characterized across different intersectional social locations based on individual-level data on social identities or social positions (e.g., Agénor et al. 2019; Cairney et al. 2014), providing groups with information on their health and potentially allowing for more precise public health interventions. A range of statistical and machine learning methods exist for this type of data analysis, though some methods produce more accurate intersection-specific outcome estimates (Mahendran et al. 2022b, 2022a).

While such approaches offer a more refined mapping of health inequalities, one limitation is that like gendered racial microaggressions, some constructs cannot be measured across intersections. Inter-categorical approaches require that constructs have similar meanings, and in research can be measured with similar validity, across groups (Bauer and Scheim 2019a; Harnois and Bastos 2019; Jackson and VanderWeele 2019). This requires careful consideration of how even common constructs such as depressive symptoms, family functioning, thriving, or social support may have different meanings across intersections. Differential meanings may create misinterpretations in research and mistargeted or inappropriate public health strategies in health promotion or education.

Inter-categorical approaches, like intra-categorical approaches, are not limited to describing experiences. In public health research, moving beyond comparison and assessment of inequalities in level or prevalence and toward causally oriented studies of drivers of inequity, is important if we are to identify modifiable factors to improve equity (Bauer 2014; Bauer and Scheim 2019b). Intra-categorical and inter-categorical approaches can also be combined in study design and analysis (Wesson et al. 2021) and in the design structure, survey instruments, and team processes of large studies (Scheim et al. 2023). Such approaches allow for consideration of intersection-specific factors that may impact health, as well as for comparison.

Another core idea of intersectionality, *social context*, is required for a full intersectional conceptualization and interpretation and is necessary to remediate public health's historic focus on individual behavior and biology as isolated factors largely independent of context. Social context can be brought into conceptualizations through intersectional understandings of what Collins terms the matrix of domination, the interlocking systems of social power that shape experiences and opportunities in life—and of course health (Collins 1990). Commonly used social-ecological models that position individual factors within concentric circles of group and social factors will help contextualize an individual-level understanding of health behavior, biology, or health services access. Recent work on structural discrimination shows how power functions through social context and is often implicitly intersectional—for example, in the ways that racism is entwined with sex/gender and economics in policy-shaped housing patterns. Public health research has only recently begun to include method work on structural racism (Adkins-Jackson et al. 2022; Bailey et al. 2021), structural sexism (Homan 2019), structural ableism (Lundberg and Chen 2024), and structural transphobia, biphobia, and homophobia (Sell and Krims 2021). Further work on structural discrimination may more explicitly advance intersectional conceptualizations.

Finally, intersectionality is about praxis as well as conceptualization (Collins 2015; Collins and Bilge 2020). It has been noted that intersectionality works well with community-based participatory research (CBPR) approaches in public health (Agénor 2020), and this may be particularly true for intra-categorical approaches to the specificity of experience. In particular, where a social intersection of interest matches up with individual and community identity, CBPR provides an opportunity to work within the community to make their experiences visible in research-informed settings and to inform health promotion and education work, as well as other interventions. Intersectionality's focus on social power challenges us to deepen our practice with regard to membership, power, and decision-making on public health education and research teams and in the healthcare systems.

Common Misconceptions: What is Intersectionality Not?

Intersectionality is *not about identity per se*. It is about social status and social power, which may at times be related to identity. "Identity" is sometimes used as a catch-all for social groups that may not constitute personal identities. One does not, for example, have to identify as poor to be affected by poverty, identify as queer or gay to be targeted by homophobic violence, or identify as Black to be targeted by anti-Black racism (Bauer 2014). The study of social identities is its own field, with consideration of identity as a developmental process, as well as the multidimensionality of identity centrality, identity salience, and other aspects of identity and community connection (Ashmore et al. 2004). In intersectionality, we are interested in the ways social power plays out across differences in social status or position and how it is entwined in meaning and structure and affects group experiences and outcomes.

Intersectionality is *not the consideration of multiple social identities or positions, or even multiple social marginalizations*. These can be studied using other non-intersectional frameworks, such as a social determinants of health approach. One can study racism and sexism, for example, and do so in a way that is not intersectional. It is important to note that this was the foundational legal conceptualization that Crenshaw brought to intersectionality when she gave it this name. Crenshaw drew on the civil rights case *Degraffenreid v. General Motors* to illustrate how having rights protected under grounds of both race and sex failed to protect Black women (Crenshaw 1989). Essentially, General Motors was determined in court not to have discriminated against Black women because they hired women (White women in the offices) and Black people (Black men on the shop floor). Did this hiring of "women" (thus no sex discrimination) and "Black people" (thus no racial discrimination) imply that there were job opportunities for Black women, who were ostensibly members of both groups? Not in the least.

Finally, intersectionality is *not an assumption or hypothesis about outcomes*. In particular, it is not the hypothesis that if group A has it bad and group B has it bad, then someone who is a member of both groups has it extra bad. In research terms, it is not the assumption of a synergistic interaction along axes of social marginalization.

Bringing Privilege into Intersectional Understandings of Marginalization

While intersectional scholarship has focused most heavily on relationality across multiple marginalizations, this may in part reflect an earlier emergence of intersectionality within qualitative studies. Such studies are often intra-categorical and thus require labor-intensive data collection and analysis that limit the number of intersections studied. Thus, this approach has reflected the need to prioritize those most marginalized. However, few people live out their lives in exclusively marginalized social locations, and exploring the ways that privileges and marginalizations interact relationally is possible within both qualitative and quantitative research models. The growth of quantitative public health research taking an explicitly intersectional approach provides opportunities for exploring health disparities across a larger number of inter-sections, including those that combine privileges and marginalizations in differing ways (Bauer 2014).

Questions of how privilege may function differently in combination with different marginalizations, or how multiple privileges may function together in interdependent ways provide an opportunity for a deeper understanding of the forces that shape health inequity. Incorporation of understandings of privilege and intersectionality into a growing understanding of stigma and discrimination has the potential to improve our understanding of how contemporary and historical power structures shape the public's health and to better identify opportunities for improvement.

References

Adkins-Jackson, Paris B., Tongtan Chantarat, Zinzi D. Bailey, and Ninez A. Ponce. 2022. "Measuring Structural Racism: A Guide for Epidemiologists and Other Health Researchers." *American Journal of Epidemiology* 191 (4): 539–547.

Agénor, Madina. 2020. "Future Directions for Incorporating Intersectionality into Quantitative Population Health Research." *American Journal of Public Health* 110 (6): 803–806.

Agénor, Madina, Ashley E. Pérez, Jonathan Wyatt Koma, Jasmine A. Abrams, Alecia J. McGregor, and Bisola O. Ojikutu. 2019. "Sexual Orientation Identity,

Race/Ethnicity, and Lifetime HIV Testing in a National Probability Sample of US Women and Men: An Intersectional Approach." *LGBT Health* 6 (6): 306–318.

Ashmore, Richard D., Kay Deaux, and Tracy McLaughlin-Volpe. 2004. "An Organizing Framework for Collective Identity: Articulation and Significance of Multidimensionality." *Psychological Bulletin* 130 (1): 80.

Bailey, Zinzi D., Justin M. Feldman, and Mary T. Bassett. 2021. "How Structural Racism Works: Racist Policies as a Root Cause of US Racial Health Inequities." *New England Journal of Medicine* 384 (8): 768–773.

Bauer, Greta R. 2014. "Incorporating Intersectionality Theory into Population Health Research Methodology: Challenges and the Potential to Advance Health Equity." *Social Science & Medicine* 110: 10–17.

Bauer, Greta R., Siobhan M. Churchill, Mayuri Mahendran, Chantel Walwyn, Daniel Lizotte, and Alma Angelica Villa-Rueda. 2021. "Intersectionality in Quantitative Research: A Systematic Review of Its Emergence and Applications of Theory and Methods." *SSM Population Health* 14: 100798.

Bauer, Greta R., and Ayden I. Scheim. 2019a. "Advancing Quantitative Intersectionality Research Methods: Intracategorical and Intercategorical Approaches to Shared and Differential Constructs." *Social Science & Medicine* 226: 260–262.

Bauer, Greta R., and Ayden I. Scheim. 2019b. "Methods for Analytic Intercategorical Intersectionality in Quantitative Research: Discrimination as a Mediator of Health Inequalities." *Social Science & Medicine* 226: 236–245.

Bello, Barbara Giovanna, and Letizia Mancini. 2016. "Talking about Intersectionality. Interview with Kimberlé W. Crenshaw." *Sociologia del Diritto* 2: 11–21.

Bowleg, Lisa. 2008. "When Black + Lesbian + Woman ≠ Black Lesbian Woman: The Methodological Challenges of Qualitative and Quantitative Intersectionality Research." *Sex Roles* 59: 312–325.

Bowleg, Lisa. 2012. "The Problem with the Phrase Women and Minorities: Intersectionality: An Important Theoretical Framework for Public Health." *American Journal of Public Health* 102 (7): 1267–1273.

Bowleg, Lisa. 2013. "'Once You've Blended the Cake, You Can't Take the Parts Back to the Main Ingredients': Black Gay and Bisexual Men's Descriptions and Experiences of Intersectionality." *Sex Roles* 68: 754–767.

Bowleg, Lisa, and Greta Bauer. 2016. "Invited Reflection: Quantifying Intersectionality." *Psychology of Women Quarterly* 40 (3): 337–341.

Cairney, John, Scott Veldhuizen, Simone Vigod, David L. Streiner, Terrance J. Wade, and Paul Kurdyak. 2014. "Exploring the Social Determinants of Mental Health Service Use Using Intersectionality Theory and CART Analysis." *Journal of Epidemiol Community Health* 68 (2)): 145–150.

Canadian Institutes of Health Research, Institute of Gender and Health, and G. Bauer. 2021. "Quantitative Intersectional Study Design and Primary Data Collection"

Meet the Methods Series, CIHR Institute of Gender and Health. https://cihr-irsc. gc.ca/e/documents/intersectional-study-design-data-collection_EN.pdf.

Canadian Institutes of Health Research, Institute of Gender and Health, H. Pruden, and T. Salway. (2020). "What and Who is 'Two-Spirit' in Health Research" Meet the Methods Series, CIHR Institute of Gender and Health. https://cihr-irsc.gc.ca/ e/documents/igh_two_spirit-en.pdf.

Cho, Sumi K., Kimberlé Williams Crenshaw, and Leslie McCall. 2013. "Toward a Field of Intersectionality Studies: Theory, applications, and praxis". *Signs*, 38 (4), 785–810. https://doi.org/10.1086/669608.

Cole, Elizabeth R. 2009. "Intersectionality and Research in Psychology." *American Psychologist* 64 (3): 170–180.

Collins, Patricia Hill. 2015. "Intersectionality's Definitional Dilemmas." *Annual Review of Sociology* 41: 1–20.

Collins, Patricia Hill. 2022. *Black Feminist Thought: Knowledge, Consciousness, and the Politics of Empowerment.* Routledge.

Collins, P. H. 2019. "Relationality within Intersectionality." *Intersectionality as Critical Social Theory* (2019): 225–252.

Collins, P. H., and S. Bilge. 2020. Intersectionality, 2nd ed. John Wiley & Sons.

Combahee River Collective. 1977. Combahee River Collective Statement. https:// americanstudies.yale.edu/sites/default/files/files/Keyword%20Coalition_ Readings.pdf.

Crenshaw, K. 1989. "Demarginalizing the Intersection of Race and Sex: A Black Feminist Critique of Antidiscrimination Doctrine, Feminist Theory and Antiracist Politics." *University of Chicago Legal Forum* 1: 139–168.

Crenshaw, K. 1991. "Mapping the Margins: Intersectionality, Identity Politics, and Violence against Women of Color." *Stanford Law Review* 42 (6): 1241–1300.

Davis, A. Y. 1983. *Women, Race & Class*, 1st ed. Vintage.

Evans, Clare R., David R. Williams, Jukka-Pekka Onnela, and S. V. Subramanian. 2018. "A Multilevel Approach to Modeling Health Inequalities at the Intersection of Multiple Social Identities." *Social Science & Medicine* 203: 64–73.

Guan, Alice, Marilyn Thomas, Eric Vittinghoff, Lisa Bowleg, Christina Mangurian, and Paul Wesson. 2021. "An Investigation of Quantitative Methods for Assessing Intersectionality in Health Research: A Systematic Review." *SSM Population Health* 16: 100977.

Hancock, Ange-Marie. 2007. "When Multiplication Doesn't Equal Quick Addition: Examining Intersectionality as a Research Paradigm." *Perspectives on Politics* 5 (1): 63–79.

Harnois, Catherine E., and João L. Bastos. 2019. "The Promise and Pitfalls of Intersectional Scale Development." *Social Science & Medicine* 223: 73–76.

Homan, Patricia. 2019. "Structural Sexism and Health in the United States: A New Perspective on Health Inequality and the Gender System." *American Sociological Review* 84 (3): 486–516.

Iezzoni, Lisa I., Amy J. Wint, Suzanne C. Smeltzer, and Jeffrey L. Ecker. 2015. "'How Did That Happen?' Public Responses to Women with Mobility Disability During Pregnancy." *Disability and Health Journal* 8 (3): 380–387.

Jackson, John W., and Tyler J. VanderWeele. 2019. "Intersectional Decomposition Analysis with Differential Exposure, Effects, and Construct." *Social Science & Medicine* 226: 254–259.

Jacobs, Sue-Ellen, Wesley Thomas, and Sabine Lang, eds. 1997. *Two-Spirit People: Native American Gender Identity, Sexuality, and Spirituality*. University of Illinois Press.

Keum, Brian TaeHyuk, Jennifer L. Brady, Rajni Sharma, Yun Lu, Young Hwa Kim, and Christina J. Thai. 2018. "Gendered Racial Microaggressions Scale for Asian American Women: Development and Initial Validation." *Journal of Counseling Psychology* 65 (5): 571.

Lewis, Jioni A., and Helen A. Neville. 2015. "Construction and Initial Validation of the Gendered Racial Microaggressions Scale for Black Women." *Journal of Counseling Psychology* 62 (2): 289.

Lundberg, Dielle J., and Jessica A. Chen. 2024. "Structural Ableism in Public Health and Healthcare: A Definition and Conceptual Framework." *Lancet Regional Health–Americas* 30: 100650.

Mahendran, Mayuri, Daniel Lizotte, and Greta R. Bauer. 2022a. "Describing Intersectional Health Outcomes: An Evaluation of Data Analysis Methods." *Epidemiology* 33 (3): 395–405.

Mahendran, Mayuri, Daniel Lizotte, and Greta R. Bauer. 2022b. "Quantitative Methods for Descriptive Intersectional Analysis with Binary Health Outcomes." *SSM Population Health* 17: 101032.

Mawhinney, Janet Lee. 1998. "Giving Up the Ghost, Disrupting the (Re) Production of White Privilege in Anti-Racist Pedagogy and Organizational Change." https://tspace.library.utoronto.ca/handle/1807/12096

McCall, L. 2005. The Complexity of Intersectionality. *Signs: Journal of Women in Culture and Society* 30 (3): 1771–1800.

McIntosh, Peggy. 2019. "White privilege: Unpacking the invisible knapsack (1989)." *On Privilege, Fraudulence, and Teaching as Learning: Selected Essays 1981–2019.* Routledge.

Misra, Joya, Celeste Vaughan Curington, and Venus Mary Green. 2021. "Methods of Intersectional Research." *Sociological Spectrum* 41 (1): 9–28.

Quillian, Lincoln, Devah Pager, Ole Hexel, and Arnfinn H. Midtbøen. 2017. "Meta-Analysis of Field Experiments Shows No Change in Racial Discrimination in

Hiring Over Time." *Proceedings of the National Academy of Sciences* 114 (41): 10870–10875.

Scheim, A. I., H. Santos, S. Ciavarella, J. Vermilion, F. S. E. Arps, N. Adams, K. Nation, & G. R. Bauer. 2023. "Intersecting inequalities in access to justice for trans and non-binary sex workers in Canada". *Sexuality Research and Social Policy* 20 (3), 1245–1257. https://doi.org/10.1007/s13178-023-00795-2

Sell, R. L., & E. I. Krims. 2021. "Structural transphobia, homophobia, and biphobia in public health practice: The example of COVID-19 surveillance". *American Journal of Public Health*, 111 (9), 1620–1626. https://doi.org/10.2105/AJPH.2021.306277

Stuber, J., I. Meyer, & B. Link. 2008. "Stigma, prejudice, discrimination and health". *Social Science & Medicine*, 67 (3), 351–357. https://doi.org/10.1016/j.socscimed.2008.03.023

Tuck, E., & K. W. Yang. 2012. "Decolonization is not a metaphor". *Decolonization: Indigeneity, Education & Society*, 1 (1), 1–40.

Wesson, P., E. Vittinghoff, C. Turner, S. Arayasirikul, W. McFarland, & E. Wilson. 2021. "Intercategorical and intracategorical experiences of discrimination and HIV prevalence among transgender women in San Francisco, CA: A quantitative intersectionality analysis". *American Journal of Public Health*, 111(3), 446–456. https://doi.org/10.2105/AJPH.2020.306055

Chapter 7

Race Theories, Antiracism, and Applications for Health

Sharon D. Jones-Eversley

Introduction

Race theories provide a cultural context and stimulate intersectional research pathways in which race and race-related aspects, knowledge, and understanding are elevated, debated, and birthed. Critical race theory is a race theory that posits that the sociopolitical construction of race privileges White Americans while it dehumanizes and discriminates against non-White people, particularly Black people (Bhopal 2023). This chapter will review critical race theory, the various levels at which racism operates in public health, and how public health has been complicit in racist structures. The chapter also uses race as a social construct and the critical race theory and racial trauma theory as lenses that explain why the medical science and public health contributions of Black scientists like Rebecca Lee Crumpler, Mary Eliza Mahoney, W. E. B. Du Bois, and James McCune Smith during the Progressive Era were suppressed or whitewashed.

The critical race theory and racial trauma theory serve as foundational theories to advocate for antiracism in public health. The chapter will end by presenting two methodology approaches: culturally responsive and equitable evaluation (CREE) and decolonizing research methodological approaches. Both methodological approaches align with the critical race theory and racial trauma theory. Collectively, the methodologies and theories may result in promising antiracist health education, practices, and research that can systematically benefit marginalized and minoritized populations.

Sharon D. Jones-Eversley, *Race Theories, Antiracism, and Applications for Health*. In: *Power, Privilege, and Public Health in the United States*. Edited by: Lorraine T. Dean and Keilah A. Jacques, Oxford University Press.

Critical Race Theory and Race Trauma Theory: Equitable Lenses to Explore Antiracism

Antiracism is a human-affirming and ongoing commitment that supports the racial identity and racial equity in a multicultural society. Antiracism actively opposes racism and the dehumanization of historically oppressed and socially suppressed racial and ethnic groups (Hassen et al. 2021; Kendi 2019). To ensure summative accountability and real reforms in public health globally, antiracism ideology and commitments to racial justice must be real, robust, and permanent (Rahman-Shepherd et al. 2023). This chapter uses two race theories, the critical race theory and the race trauma theory, to identify and advocate for antiracism in public health research, education, and practice.

Critical race theory is the preferred framework to identify historical and current power and privilege operative in the public health field in the US (Delgado and Stefancic 2005). By highlighting public health's systemic racist aspects and antiracist potential, the critical race theory (CRT) examines race and racism in public health and the CRT's ability to assist in better understanding how public health can incite either health disparities or health equities. Though viewed by some as politically divisive and polarizing, the CRT has and continues to be used as a humanizing lens to assess the intersectionality of racial inequality and educational, social, legal, political, ethnic, and oppressive characteristics in the United States (Berman et al. 2023; Delgado and Stefancic 2023).

Like the CRT, the racial trauma theory (RTT) is also an equitable lens to explore antiracism in public health. The racial trauma theory is an ethical response to social justice that identifies antiracism and addresses racist and oppressive systemic institutions and practices (Mosley et al. 2021). Additionally, the racial trauma theory illuminates the race-based traumatic and internalized racist social practices many racially marginalized and minoritized people of color, such as Black people, may experience in racist and oppressive spaces and institutions (Cénat 2023; Comas-Díaz et al. 2019). The persistent societal racism and psychosocial stresses are weathering and prematurely killing Black people at alarming near-epidemic rates (Beech et al. 2021; Geronimus 1992). Antiracist public health education, research, and practice may be the ideal societal and humane antidotes that America needs to cease its historically racist-accommodating and dehumanization-tolerating public health system.

In light of the alarming resurgence of overt and covert racism in the US, the health equity intents of public health are severely jeopardized if race and racism are not finally addressed and resolved (Bracke and Aguilar 2024). Thus, antiracism must be infused and homogenized in public health education, research, and practice. W. E. B. Du Bois is justifiably the father of social epidemiology (Jones-Eversley and Dean 2018), and he predicted that if the US's race and racism challenges were not addressed and resolved, they would become and remain generational problems for the country (Du Bois 1903/1899). Therefore, due to Black people's historical, consistent, and disproportionate health inequities and high mortality, morbidity, disability, and racial trauma rates, this chapter will highlight Black people and their health as both a racially marginalized and minoritized subgroup (Krumholz et al. 2022; Phelan and Link 2015). The poor health outcomes, racism, and health disparities of Black people were evident even during the trans-Atlantic slave trade (Kiple and Kiple 1980). Through the posttraumatic slave syndrome, intergenerationally cultural trauma continues to impact Black people and their health (Degruy-Leary 2017; Halloran 2019; Kiple and Kiple 1980).

Race, Racism, Dehumanization, and Whitewashing of Black People in Public Health

Race and racism intersect, but they are not synonymous. Race is viewed as a status stratification, not a biological construct. This chapter operationalizes race as an artificial social construct based on skin pigmentation, intellectual assumptions, privileged access or denial, and physical appearance (Fitzgerald 2023; Wijeysinghe et al. 1997). Racism is a structural subordination and racialized dogma that fictitiously labels, overtly and covertly, targeted racial groups as inferior, marginalized, and void of social dominance (Bonilla-Silva 1997; Wijeysinghe et al. 1997).

The dehumanization of Black people in public health stems from the deeply embedded anti-Blackness beliefs and practices that commenced during US colonial history (Paine et al. 2021). As a revolt against Europe's hierarchy-based systems of dehumanization, classism, and imperialism, America was deliberately founded on anti-imperialism and social equity principles of freedom, humanity, justice, civil liberties, and human rights. However, America's fundamental human rights were selectively privileged to only naturalized White people (Paik 2023). The colonists did not consider the enslaved Africans they kidnapped to be humans (Okoye 1980). They viewed the Black Africans they enslaved as chattel void of souls and human rights (Buhring 2022; Mitchell 1999). Politically, socially, and medically, America legalized and legitimized a race-based chattel system that enslaved, exploited, mischaracterized, experimented on, brutalized, and dehumanized Black people and their bodies (Goff et al. 2008; Jardina and Piston 2023).

A pivotal yet structured facet of the dehumanization of Black people in America is whitewashing historical references that deny the terrorizing and traumatic truths of the enslavement of Black people (Brown et al. 2023; Kern 2024). The current backlash about the CRT is a racist, systemic, and targeted instance of whitewashing. In 2020, CRT attracted controversy after a presidential executive order banned curricula rooted in critical race theory for federal workers and contractors (Filimon and Ivănescu 2024; Hamilton 2021). Whitewashing denies America's historical and inhumane actualities, and it aims to delete the legalized brutality of enslaved Africans and Black people (Fowler 2023).

The enslavement and dehumanization of Black people is a part of American history and its public health history. Public health education, research, and practices should acknowledge the enslavement and dehumanization of Black people and resist the complicity of whitewashing and erasing it (Wright 2002). Current and next-generation public health researchers, educators, practitioners, and professionals should know historical facts and racist assumptions about the flawed research that dehumanized Black people.

American anthropologist Carleton S. Coon's flawed scientific research is an example of the dehumanization of Black people. Coon's research affirmed that Black people, whom he referred to as Negroid, were inferior species and White people, classified as Caucasoid, Mongolid, and Australoid, as superior species (Jackson 2001). Additionally, the global eugenics movement, a racist theory led by White scientists, perpetuated the false social hierarchical narrative that supported the procreation and inclusion of "superior" humans and the exclusion and sterilization of "inferior" humans (Barrett and Kurzman 2004).

Even though the eugenics movement's flawed science considered Black people biologically inferior, modern-day "Whiteness studies scholars" hypothesize that during slavery, White people had poorer outcomes than enslaved Black people (Reece 2019; Okeagu et. al. 2010). Eugenics' racist and dehumanizing scientific research should be taught and reevaluated through scientifically sound and antiracist lenses. Even though racist scientific claims of inferiority, stereotypes, and dehumanization of people of color were debunked by multiple scientists in the 1950s, public health, like countless other science-led fields, disregarded the discrediting of the research and, instead, clung to the pluralistic racial ignorance that perpetuated the racist research and white supremacist ideologies (Kirkland 2021; White et al. 2021). This dangerous practice among scientists, scholars, and researchers led to centuries of hateful racial discourse that ignored Black health scholars, intellectual forerunners, and theorists while still dehumanizing Black people and their bodies in the US.

To counter the flawed eugenics research studies of the Progressive Era with antiracist applications, public health researchers, educators, and practitioners must leverage the suppressed and whitewashed medical science and public health contributions of Black scientists, researchers, and practitioners like Dr. Rebecca Lee Crumpler, Nurse Mary Eliza Mahoney, Dr. W. E. B. Du Bois, and Dr. James McCune Smith.

In 1864, Dr. Rebecca Lee Crumpler was the first Black woman to earn a medical degree in the US. She graduated from New England Female Medical College. Dr. Crumpler was a forerunner in US maternal and child health practice and research, but few scientists, medical doctors, and researchers have been taught about her contributions (Brown 2023). Due to the prevailing and alarming US Black maternal, Black infant, and Black child morbidity and mortality rates, an in-depth analysis of her work would be an example of antiracism-affirming practices in public health (Clare et al. 2020).

Also, the Civil War era was an intensely dangerous and violent time for Black people. The RTT would be an interesting theory to use to examine the kinds of racist and traumatic challenges Dr. Crumpler may have experienced in her life and profession. For over 160 years, Dr. Crumpler's contributions to public health were whitewashed from public health and medical pedagogy, research, and publications. Acknowledging Dr. Crumpler's contributions to medicine and public health is a powerful societal and humanizing antidote that further elevates antiracist research, education, and practice.

While Mary Eliza Mahoney's contributions to nursing are more widely known than Dr. Rebecca Lee Crumpler's, Mary Eliza Mahoney's historic role in nursing must always be humanized and never whitewashed (Chayer 1954). In 1879, she was the first Black licensed nurse in the US (Coles 1969). She was an avid believer in equity, particularly for Black people and women. She was the cofounder of the National Association of Colored Graduate Nurses (Chayer 1954). It would be worthwhile to use the CRT to explore Mahoney's historic accomplishments and compare them to the emerging role of nurse practitioners in the US. The comparison analysis could help emphasize the systemic dangers of whitewashing public health history. Also, increasing the number of Black, Indigenous, and people of color (BIPOC) in the nursing field is another way to homogenize antiracist research, education, and practice in public health (Montgomery et al. 2021; Sanford 2020).

The CRT and RTT are equitable lenses that highlight Dr. W. E. B. Du Bois's contributions in public health. In 1895, he was the first Black person to earn a Ph.D. from Harvard University. His decolonizing sociology and critical sociology research perspectives and the intersectional lenses he utilized in examining racism in health were and remain groundbreaking (Burawoy 2021; Jones-Eversley and Dean 2018). The eugenics movement's flawed research studies that deemed Black people are inferior were debunked by Dr. Du Bois during the Progressive Era. In his mixed-methodology research, the Philadelphia Negro Study, Dr. Du Bois identified the health disparities in the US. His study meticulously examined the social, political, environmental, and economic structural factors contributing to the US's high mortality and morbidity rates (Du Bois and Eaton 1995).

Unfortunately, in the US, white supremacy ideologies muted Dr. Du Bois's public health contributions, and Dr. Du Bois and his scholarly works were whitewashed from US medical and public health publications. Therefore, it would be interesting to have current and future public health students write a "reimagined" research paper on how current-day health outcomes, healthcare, and antiracist public health in the US could have been different if Dr. Du Bois's scientific research methodologies had not been suppressed and whitewashed for over a century.

Like Rebecca Lee Crumpler, Mary Eliza Mahoney, and W. E. B. Du Bois, Dr. James McCune Smith made history in the US. He was the first Black physician to hold a medical degree in the US (Smith 2006). However, Dr. Smith earned his medical degree with honors from the University of Glasgow in Scotland. He was denied admission to Geneva Medical College and Columbia University in New York. Had the racist elements of the dehumanization of Black people not existed in the US, Dr. Smith would have been accepted into US medical colleges (Aggarwal 2021; Hansen 1984; Lujan and DiCarlo 2019).

The powerful irony of his brilliance and resilience is that Dr. Smith was born into slavery in New York in 1813. New York freed enslaved Black people in 1827, so at the age of fourteen, he was no longer enslaved. But sadly, in 1865, he died in New York just weeks before the federal Emancipation Proclamation Act was ratified (Lujan and DiCarlo 2019; Lynerd and Wartell 2023). Dr. Smith was a physician, author, researcher, and abolitionist. He is the epitome of what antiracist public health educators, researchers, and professionals should strive to be and become.

Because he was the first Black person to publish his research in US medical journals, a thought-provoking antiracist assignment for medical and public health students would be to write literature reviews of his scientific methods and publications and to compare them with eugenic scientists like Charles Darwin, Carleton S. Coon, Carl Vogt, Samuel George Morton, and

Samuel Cartwright (Morgan 2005; Quintyn 2023; Rupke 2018; Slorach 2020; Willoughby 2018).

White Supremacy Conspiracies Threaten Public Health Antiracism Efforts

Even though the American Public Health Association has acknowledged racism as a public health crisis, and the American Anthropological Association vehemently censured racism and biological essentialism, the American nationalist views of the modern-day revisionist theory of racism have revitalized white supremacy ideologies (Urquidez 2020; Wu et al. 2023; Zack 2001). White-body power, White-body privilege, White-body social dominance, and white supremacy ideologies have heightened popularity in the US. White nationalists are promoting the great replacement conspiracy (Obaidi et al. 2022). The great replacement conspiracy poses a threat to the health and lives of Black people because the conspiracy aims to reject the history and lived experiences of racially marginalized people (Chamie 2022). The inhumane captivity of enslaved Africans during the Atlantic slave trade and the ongoing societal dehumanization of Black bodies and their lives have resulted in inaccurate racial assumptions, unjust treatment, poor health outcomes, and health disparities among Black people (Curtin 1968; Kirland 2021; Kwate and Meyer 2011). Unfortunately, White-body power, White-body privilege, White-body social dominance, and white supremacy ideologies perpetuate racial trauma, and they remain an existential threat to the racially marginalized and minoritized in the US (Matthew 2024). Perilous racial discourse poses either a pragmatic risk to diminish public health antiracist efforts or serves as an opportunity to elevate public health's antiracism agenda progressively.

In 2020, during the contentious racial discourse in the US, the American Medical Association acknowledged that race is not an inherent risk for disease (American Medical Association 2020). Its policy goals were to dismantle the racial misconceptions in healthcare and public health. Despite the AMA's antiracist attempts to end racial essentialism, Black people, Black bodies, and their health have not always been humanized in public health education, research, and practices (Flanagin et al. 2021). Hence, designing culturally responsive and equitable educational curricula and healthcare environments that institutionalize antiracist public health education, practice, and research is essential to affirm Black people's humanization and human rights for equitable health (Royal 2023; Webb and Pérez-Stable 2023).

Systematically homogenizing antiracist public health education, practices, and research, pedagogical modules must resist the social and political pressures of whitewashing Black scientists, practitioners, and professionals from history. The public health acknowledgments of Rebecca Lee Crumpler, Mary Eliza Mahoney, W. E. B. Du Bois, and James McCune Smith must never be suppressed again. Likewise, in research studies published during the slavery era, the studies' internal and external validity should be reassessed by current and future medical and public health students (Andrade 2018). Perhaps looking through an epidemiological lens, students could review enslaved African cargo's morbidity and mortality data from the insurance companies who sold and curated the records during the transatlantic slave trade era (Chen and Simon 2004; Farber 2023).

Medical and public health students could also use the epidemiological triangle to examine the host, vector, environment, and persons harmed. In addition to assessing the insurance companies' morbidity and mortality data, students could compare the leading causes of death of enslaved Black people to the current leading causes of death among Black people. These antiracist research exercises may educate current and next-generation researchers and epidemiologists in the importance of assessing data from a human and health perspective that is sanitized of racist assumptions of Black inferiority and whitewashing (Adkins-Jackson et al. 2022).

Conclusion

In the US, racism and White supremacy are social germs, and like any dangerous pathogens, once transmitted by humans to other humans, racism and White supremacy could harm, traumatize, disable, or kill others (Jones-Eversley and Dean 2018) (Figure 7.1).The dehumanization of Black people in public health can no longer be tolerated. Current and future public health students, professors, and researchers should continuously be trained in racial equity and health equity (Chandler et al. 2022; Gould et al. 2023).

The historical racist public health applications of imperialism, the dehumanization of Black people, and White supremacy have and continue to compromise the health and well-being of Black people in the US. This chapter offered several antiracist and humanity-affirming recommendations for public health education, research, and practice. Also, exploring culturally responsive and equitable evaluation (CREE) and decolonizing research methodology approaches should become priorities in public health.

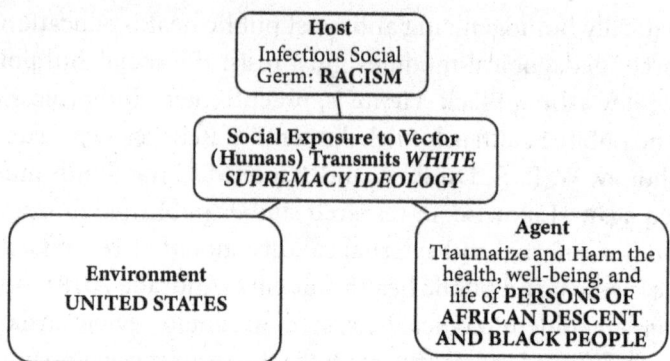

Figure 7.1 The pathology of racism and White supremacy through the epidemiological triangle. The epidemiological triangle illustrates the social germ of racism and how humans who believe and exemplify the ideology of White supremacy could knowingly or unknowingly serve as vectors that socially infect others and transmit and direct their racism to persons of African descent and Black people in the US.
Source: Figure conceptualized and designed by the author.

According to Expanding the Bench, the CREE research methodology approach integrates diversity, inclusion, and equity in all research and evaluation phases (Expanding the Bench Team and Advisory Team 2019). The goal of CREE is to elevate the awareness of racism and promote antiracist research and evaluation. By design, CREE's antiracist principles make racial equity, people's lived experiences, historical relevance, and their social norms acknowledged and valued throughout all research and evaluation phases (Fort et al. 2023). CREE is being increasingly used in public health research, community participatory research, program development, and program planning (Kushnier et al. 2023).

The decolonizing research methodological approaches also provide antiracist aspects that may aid in deconstructing past, current, and future racial biases and assumptions about marginalized and minoritized people, their health, and their bodies. Decolonizing methodologies also prioritize the cultural and social norms and history of the lived experiences of people, particularly Indigenous people (Smith 2021). Decolonizing research methodologies dismantle the Eurocentric research methods' role; instead, it leverages the research methodologies and processes unique to and identified by the Indigenous population being researched (Keikelame and Swartz 2019).

The CREE-informed and decolonizing research methodologies are needed approaches in public health curricula, interdisciplinary training modalities, and antiracist programming and practices that are key to normalizing

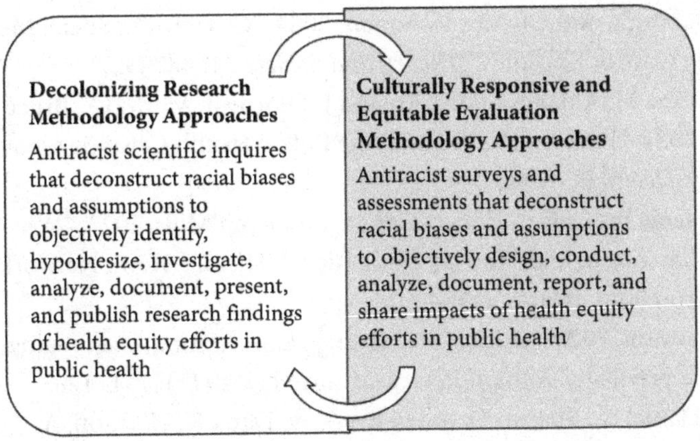

Figure 7.2 Decolonizing research and culturally responsive and equitable evaluation methodological approaches. The figure highlights the complementary aspects of two antiracist methodological approaches that could be used in public health education, research, and practice.

Source: Figure conceptualized and designed by the author.

equity-centered public health education and research (Keikelame and Swartz 2019; Lee et al. 2023; Tsai 2022) (Figure 7.2).

In conclusion, by utilizing CRT, RTT, and CREE and decolonizing research methodologies, public health research has the potential to decompose the existing racist and dehumanizing research, education, and practices and transform it into an antiracist and humanizing practicing (Naidu et al. 2023).

References

Adkins-Jackson, Paris B., Tongtan Chantarat, Zinzi D. Bailey, and Ninez A. Ponce. 2022. "Measuring Structural Racism: A Guide for Epidemiologists and Other Health Researchers." *American Journal of Epidemiology* 191 (4): 539–547.

Aggarwal N. K. 2021. "The Legacy of James McCune Smith, MD: The First US Black Physician." *Journal of the American Medical Association* 326 (22): 2245–2246.

American Medical Association. 2020. "New AMA Policies Recognize Race as a Social, Not Biological, Construct." Press release. https://www.ama-assn.org/press-center/press-releases/new-amapolicies-recognize-race-social-not-biological-construct. Accessed August 10, 2021.

Andrade, Chittaranjan. 2018. "Internal, External, and Ecological Validity in Research Design, Conduct, and Evaluation." *Indian Journal of Psychological Medicine* 40 (5): 498–499.

Barrett, Deborah, and Charles Kurzman. 2004. "Globalizing Social Movement Theory: The Case of Eugenics." *Theory and Society* 33: 487–527.

Beech, Bettina M., Chandra Ford, Roland J. Thorpe Jr, Marino A. Bruce, and Keith C. Norris. 2021. "Poverty, Racism, and the Public Health Crisis in America." *Frontiers in Public Health* 9: 699049.

Berman, Stacie Brensilver, Robert Cohen, and Ryan Mills. 2023. "Why CRT Belongs in the Classroom, and How to Do It Right." History News Network. January 22, 2023. http://hnn.us/article/184803.

Bhopal, Kalwant. 2023. "Critical race theory: Confronting, challenging, and rethinking white privilege." *Annual Review of Sociology* 49 (1): 111–128.

Boamah, Daniel A., Sharon D. Jones-Eversley, Dana K. Harmon, A. Christson Adedoyin, Kelsey Leann Burton, Sharon Sanders, Christopher A. Jones, Brittany J. Nwachuku, and Sharon E. Moore. 2022. "Dismantling Structural Racism and White Supremacy through Course Assignments That Integrate Faith and Learning in Social Work Curriculum." *Social Work & Christianity* 49 (1): 26–47.

Bonilla-Silva, Eduardo. 1997. "Rethinking racism: Toward a structural interpretation." *American Sociological Review*: 465–480.

Bracke, Sarah, and Luis Manuel Hernández Aguilar. 2024. "The Politics of Replacement: From "Race Suicide" to the "Great Replacement"." In *The Politics of Replacement*, pp. 1–19. Routledge.

Brown, Jasmine. 2023. *Twice as Hard: The Stories of Black Women Who Fought to Become Physicians, from the Civil War to the 21st Century*. Beacon Press.

Brown, Michael K., Martin Carnoy, Elliott Currie, Troy Duster, David B. Oppenheimer, Marjorie M. Shultz, and David Wellman. 2023. *Whitewashing Race: The Myth of a Color-Blind Society*. University of California Press.

Buhring, Kurt. 2022. "The Spirit (s) in Slavery: African American Christianity." In *Spirit(s) in Black Religion: Fire on the Inside*, pp. 99–144. Cham: Springer International Publishing.

Burawoy, Michael. 2021. "Decolonizing Sociology: The Significance of WEB Du Bois." *Critical Sociology* 47 (4–5): 545–554.

Cénat, Jude Mary. 2023. "Complex Racial Trauma: Evidence, Theory, Assessment, and Treatment." *Perspectives on Psychological Science* 18 (3): 675–687.

Chamie, Joseph. 2022. "The 'Great Replacement' Theory Rejects History and Reality." In *Population Levels, Trends, and Differentials: More Important Population Matters*, pp. 327–329. Cham: Springer Nature Switzerland.

Chandler, Caroline E., Caitlin R. Williams, Mallory W. Turner, and Meghan E. Shanahan. 2022. "Training Public Health Students in Racial/Justice and Health Equity: A Systematic Review." *Public Health Reports* 137 (2): 375–385.

Chayer, M. E. 1954. "Mary Eliza Mahoney." *The American Journal of Nursing* 54 (4): 429–431.

Chen, Cheryl Rhan-Hsin, and Gary Simon. 2004. "Actuarial Issues in Insurance on Slaves in the United States South." *Journal of African American History* 89 (4): 348–357.

Clare, Camille A., Ellana Stinson, and Rachel Villanueva. 2020. "What Have We Learned from Dr. Rebecca Lee Crumpler: A Commentary." *Journal of the National Medical Association* 112 (5): S23.

Coles, Anna B. 1969. "The Howard University School of Nursing in Historical Perspective." *Journal of the National Medical Association* 61 (2): 105.

Comas-Díaz, Lillian, Gordon Nagayama Hall, and Helen A. Neville. 2019. "Racial Trauma: Theory, Research, and Healing: Introduction to the Special Issue." *American Psychologist* 74 (1): 1.

Curtin, Philip D. 1968. "Epidemiology and the Slave Trade." *Political Science Quarterly* 83 (2): 190–216.

Degruy-Leary, Joy. 2017. *"Post-traumatic Slave Syndrome: America's Legacy of Enduring Injury."* Portland, OR: Joy DeGruy Publications.

Delgado, Richard, and Jean Stefancic. 2005. *"The Derrick Bell Reader: Introduction."* New York University Press.

Delgado, Richard, and Jean Stefancic. 2023. *Critical Race Theory: An Introduction.* Vol. 87. NYU Press.

Du Bois, William Edward Burghardt. 1899. *The Philadelphia Negro: A Social Study.* Published for the University.

Du Bois, W. E. B. 1903. *The Souls of Black Folk.* North Charleston, SC: Createspace Independent Publishing Platform.

Du Bois, W. E. B., & I. Eaton. 1995. *The Philadelphia Negro: A Social Study.* University of Pennsylvania Press. http://www.jstor.org/stable/j.ctt3fhpfb.

Expanding The Bench Team and Advisory Team. (2019). *History and Definition of Culturally Responsive and Equitable Evaluation.* Change Matrix. https://expandingthebench.org/cree-definition

Farber, Hannah. 2023. "Slave Trade Insurance in the Age of Abolition: Archives, Politics, and Legalities." *Slavery & Abolition* 44 (2): 350–376.

Filimon, Luiza-Maria, and Mihaela Ivănescu. 2024. "Bans, Sanctions, and Dog-Whistles: A Review of Anti-Critical Race Theory Initiatives Adopted in the United States Since 2020." *Policy Studies* 45 (2): 183–204.

Fisher, Colin. 2021. "Antebellum Black Climate Science: The Medical Geography and Emancipatory Politics of James McCune Smith and Martin Delany." *Environmental History*: 461–483.

Fitzgerald, K. J. 2023. *Recognizing race and ethnicity: Power, privilege, and inequality.* Routledge.

Flanagin, Annette, Tracy Frey, Stacy L. Christiansen, and AMA Manual of Style Committee. 2021. "Updated Guidance on the Reporting of Race and Ethnicity in Medical and Science Journals." *JAMA* 326 (7): 621–627.

Fort, Meredith P., Spero M. Manson, and Russell E. Glasgow. 2023. "Applying an Equity Lens to Assess Context and Implementation in Public Health and Health Services Research and Practice Using the PRISM Framework." *Frontiers in Health Services* 3: 1139788.

Fowler, Jermaine. 2023. *The Humanity Archive: Recovering the Soul of Black history from a Whitewashed American Myth*. Simon and Schuster.

Geronimus, Arline T. 1992. "The Weathering Hypothesis and the Health of African-American Women and Infants: Evidence and Speculations." *Ethnicity & Disease* 2(3): 207–221.

Goff, Phillip Atiba, Jennifer L. Eberhardt, Melissa J. Williams, and Matthew Christian Jackson. 2008. "Not Yet Human: Implicit Knowledge, Historical Dehumanization, and Contemporary Consequences." *Journal of Personality and Social Psychology* 94 (2): 292.

Gould, L. Hannah, Stephanie E. Farquhar, Sophia Greer, Madeline Travers, Lisa Ramadhar, L. Tantay, Danielle Gurr, et al. 2023. "Data for Equity: Creating an Antiracist, Intersectional Approach to Data in a Local Health Department." *Journal of Public Health Management and Practice* 29 (1): 11–20.

Halloran, Michael J. 2019. "African American Health and Posttraumatic Slave Syndrome: A Terror Management Theory Account." *Journal of Black Studies* 50 (1): 45–65.

Hamilton, Vivian E. 2021. "Reform, Retrench, Repeat: The Campaign against Critical Race Theory, through the Lens of Critical Race Theory." 2021. *William & Mary Journal of Race, Gender & Social Justice* 28: 61.

Hansen, Axel C. 1984. "Black Americans in Medicine." *Journal of the National Medical Association* 76 (7): 693.

Hassen, Nadha, Aisha Lofters, Sinit Michael, Amita Mall, Andrew D. Pinto, and Julia Rackal. 2021. "Implementing Anti-racism Interventions in Healthcare Settings: A Scoping Review." *International Journal of Environmental Research and Public Health* 18 (6): 2993.

Jackson, John P. 2001. "'In Ways Unacademical': The Reception of Carleton S. Coon's *The Origin of Races*." *Journal of the History of Biology* 34: 247–285.

Jardina, Ashley, and Spencer Piston. 2023. "The Politics of Racist Dehumanization in the United States." *Annual Review of Political Science* 26: 369–388.

Jones, Camara Phyllis. 2000. "Levels of Racism: A Theoretic Framework and a Gardener's Tale." *American Journal of Public Health* 90 (8): 1212.

Jones-Eversley, Sharon D., and Lorraine T. Dean. 2018. "After 121 Years, It's Time to Recognize W.E.B. Du Bois as a Founding Father of Social Epidemiology." *The Journal of Negro Education* 87 (3): 230–245.

Keikelame M. J., L. Swartz. 2019. "Decolonising research methodologies: lessons from a qualitative research project, Cape Town, South Africa". *Global Health Action*. 12 (1):1561175. doi: 10.1080/16549716.2018.1561175. PMID: 30661464; PMCID: PMC6346712.

Kendi, I. X. 2019. *How to be an antiracist*. Random House.

Kern, Emily M. 2024. "Alternate Edens: History, Evolution, and Origins in UNESCO's Cultural and Scientific History of Mankind." *Journal of the History of Ideas* 85 (1): 121–148.

Kiple, Kenneth, and Virginia Kiple. 1980. "The African Connection: Slavery, Disease and Racism." *Phylon (1960–)* 41 (3): 211–222.

Kirkland, David E. 2021. "A Pedagogy for Black People: Why Naming Race Matters." *Equity & Excellence in Education* 54 (1): 60–67.

Krumholz, Harlan M., Daisy S. Massey, and Karen B. Dorsey. 2022. "Racism as a Leading Cause of Death in the United States." BMJ 376.

Kushnier, Lauren, Shevaun Nadin, Mary Ellen Hill, Mischa Taylor, Shelly Jun, Christopher J. Mushquash, Giulia Puineanc, and Rebecca Gokiert. 2023. "Culturally Responsive Evaluation: A Scoping Review of the Evaluation Literature." *Evaluation and Program Planning* 100: 102322.

Kwate, Naa Oyo A., and Ilan H. Meyer. 2011. "ON STICKS AND STONES AND BROKEN BONES: Stereotypes and African American Health." *Du Bois Review: Social Science Research on Race* 8 (1): 191–198.

Lee, Matthew, Jake Ryann C. Sumibcay, Hannah Cory, Catherine Duarte, and Arrianna Marie Planey. 2023. "Extending Critical Race, Racialization, and Racism Literatures to the Adoption, Implementation, and Sustainability of Data Equity Policies and Data (Dis) Aggregation Practices in Health Research." *Health Services Research* 58 (Suppl 2): 262.

Lujan, Heidi L., and Stephen E. DiCarlo. 2019. "First African-American to Hold a Medical Degree: Brief History of James McCune Smith, Abolitionist, Educator, and Physician." *Advances in Physiology Education* 43 (2): 134–139.

Lynerd, Benjamin T., and Jack Wartell. 2023. "'A Natural Right to the Soil': Black Abolitionists and the Meaning of Freedom." *Journal of Black Studies* 54 (1): 62–82.

Mathew, L. (2024). Racism Is Life-Threatening and Continues the Cycle of Racial Trauma: What Can Clinicians Do to Interrupt This Cycle? *Clinical Social Work Journal* 52:265–273.

Mitchell, Michele. 1999. "'The Black Man's Burden': African Americans, Imperialism, and Notions of Racial Manhood 1890–1910." *International Review of Social History* 44 (S7): 77–99.

Montgomery, Tiffany M., J. T. Bundy, D. Cofer, and E. M. Nichols. 2021. "Black Americans in Nursing Education." *American Nurse Journal* 16 (2): 22–25.

Morgan, R. 2005. *The genetics revolution: history, fears, and future of a life-altering science.* Bloomsbury Publishing USA.

Mosley, Della V., Candice N. Hargons, Carolyn Meiller, Blanka Angyal, Paris Wheeler, Candice Davis, and Danelle Stevens-Watkins. 2021. "Critical Consciousness of Anti-Black Racism: A Practical Model to Prevent and Resist Racial Trauma." *Journal of Counseling Psychology* 68 (1): 1.

Mpoe, Johannah Keikelame, and Leslie Swartz. 2019. "Decolonising Research Methodologies: Lessons from a Qualitative Research Project, Cape Town, South Africa." *Global Health Action* 12 (1).

Naidu, Jessica, Elizabeth Oddone Paolucci, and Tanvir C. Turin. 2023. "A Critical Lens on Health: Key Principles of Critical Discourse Analysis and Its Benefits to Anti-Racism in Population Public Health Research." *Societies* 13 (2): 42.

Obaidi, Milan, Jonas Kunst, Simon Ozer, and Sasha Y. Kimel. 2022. "The 'Great Replacement' Conspiracy: How the Perceived Ousting of Whites Can Evoke Violent Extremism and Islamophobia." *Group Processes & Intergroup Relations: GPIR* 25 (7): 1675–1695.

Okoye, F. Nwabueze. 1980. "Chattel Slavery as the Nightmare of the American Revolutionaries." *The William and Mary Quarterly: A Magazine of Early American History*: 4–28.

Paik, A. Naomi. 2023. "US Imperialism and Rights." *Modern American History* 6 (1): 64–68.

Paine, Lilliann, Patanjali de la Rocha, Antonia P. Eyssallenne, Courtni Alexis Andrews, Leanne Loo, Camara Phyllis Jones, Anne Marie Collins, and Michelle Morse. 2021. "Declaring Racism a Public Health Crisis in the United States: Cure, Poison, or Both?" *Frontiers in Public Health* 9: 676784.

Pernick, Martin S. 1997. "Eugenics and Public Health in American History." *American Journal of Public Health* 87 (11): 1767–1772.

Phelan, Jo C., and Bruce G. Link. 2015. "Is Racism a Fundamental Cause of Inequalities in Health?" *Annual Review of Sociology* 41: 311–330.

Quintyn, Conrad B. 2023. "Physical Anthropology and Race: A Reckoning for the Newly Renamed 'Biological' Anthropology in 2020 and Beyond." *Journal of Sociology* 7 (1): 1–10.

Rahman-Shepherd, Afifah, Ngozi A. Erondu, Bakht Anwar, Ezekiel Boro, Thuy Duyen Chau, Renzo R. Guinto, Lara Hollmann, et al. 2023. "Antiracism in Leading Public Health Universities, Journals and Funders: Commitments, Accountability and the Decision-Makers." *BMJ Global Health* 8 (3): e010376.

Reece, Robert L. 2019. "Whitewashing Slavery: Legacy of Slavery and White Social Outcomes." *Social Problems* 67 (2): 304–323.

Royal, C. D. 2023. "Science, Society, and Dismantling Racism." *Health Equity,* 7 (1): 38–44.

Rupke, Nicolaas. 2018. "The Origins of Scientific Racism and Huxley's Rule." In *Johann Friedrich Blumenbach*, edited by Nicolaas Rupke and Gerhard Lauer, 233–247. London: Routledge.

Sanford, Kathleen D. 2020. "Always a Nurse: A Profession for a Lifetime." *Nursing Administration Quarterly* 44 (1): 4–11.

Smith, James McCune. 2006. *The Works of James McCune Smith: Black Intellectual and Abolitionist*. Oxford University Press.

Smith, Linda Tuhiwai. 2021. *Decolonizing Methodologies: Research and Indigenous Peoples*. Bloomsbury Publishing.

Slorach, R. 2020. From eugenics to scientific racism. *International Socialism Journal,* 165, 133–154.

Tsai, Jennifer. 2022. "¿ Cómo deben los educadores y editores eliminar el esencialismo racial?" *AMA Journal of Ethics* 24(3): 201–211.

United Nations Educational Scientific and Cultural Organization. 1950. "Fallacies of Racism Exposed: UNESCO Publishes Declaration by World's Scientists." *UNESCO Courier* 3 (6–7): 1–16.

Urquidez, Alberto G. 2020. "A Revisionist Theory of Racism: Rejecting the Presumption of Conservatism." *Journal of Social Philosophy* 51 (2): 231–260.

Webb Hooper, Monica, and Eliseo J. Pérez-Stable. 2023. "Health Equity Is Not Possible without Addressing Disparities." *Health Psychology* 42 (9): 625.

White, Alexandre, Rachel L. J. Thornton, and Jeremy A. Greene. 2021. "Remembering Past Lessons about Structural Racism: Recentering Black Theorists of Health and Society." *New England Journal of Medicine* 385 (9): 850–855.

Wijeyesinghe, Charmaine L., Pat Griffin, and Barbara Love. 1997. "Racism curriculum design." *Teaching for diversity and social justice: A sourcebook*: 82–109.

Williams, Richard Allen, and Richard Allen Williams. 2020. "Profiles in Courage: African American Medical Pioneers in the United States: The Earliest Black Practitioners." *Blacks in Medicine: Clinical, Demographic, and Socioeconomic Correlations*: 33–59.

Willoughby, Christopher DE. 2018. "Running Away from Drapetomania: Samuel A. Cartwright, Medicine, and Race in the Antebellum South." *Journal of Southern History* 84 (3): 579–614.

Wright, William D. 2002. *Critical Reflections on Black History*. Bloomsbury Publishing USA.

Wu, Elwin. 2023. "Health Equity Research: A Clarion Call to Focus on Racism, Not Race." *American Journal of Public Health* 113 (6): 604–606.

Zack, Naomi. 2001. "Philosophical Aspects of the 'AAA Statement on "race".'" *Anthropological Theory* 1 (4): 445–465.

Chapter 8

Why Racial Capitalism and Scientific Racism Threaten Promoting Antiracism and Health Equity in Public Health

Keon L. Gilbert and Gilbert Gee

On March 18, 2008, Barack Obama gave his "A More Perfect Union" speech, otherwise known as his "Speech on Race" in response to public criticism of his pastor, who condemned the US government for its role in racism within Black communities. Obama offered the following thoughts on how a greater sense of American community can be achieved without demoralizing or limiting access to others because of their racial, ethnic, gender, or sexual identities:

> "In the white community, the path to a more perfect union means acknowledging that what ails the African-American community does not just exist in the minds of black people; that the legacy of discrimination—and current incidents of discrimination, while less overt than in the past—are real and must be addressed, not just with words, but with deeds, by investing in our schools and our communities; by enforcing our civil rights laws and ensuring fairness in our criminal justice system; by providing this generation with ladders of opportunity that were unavailable for previous generations. It requires all Americans to realize that your dreams do not have to come at the expense of my dreams; that investing in the health, welfare and education of black and brown and white children will ultimately help all of America prosper." (Obama 2008)

Obama shared with the nation that the deep legacy of structural discrimination is not only real but has real implications for outcomes between racial groups—either positive or negative. These actions can therefore share power or limit power or even structure. The brokering of power has had inclusionary and exclusionary forces and agents. Compromises are made to ensure that representatives of power always dominate and have the tools to subjugate

Keon L. Gilbert and Gilbert Gee, *Why Racial Capitalism and Scientific Racism Threaten Promoting Antiracism and Health Equity in Public Health*. In: *Power, Privilege, and Public Health in the United States*. Edited by: Lorraine T. Dean and Keilah A. Jacques, Oxford University Press. © Oxford University Press (2025). DOI: 10.1093/9780197760956.003.0008 others. These interactions take shape across social institutions and determine the health and well-being of the nation, with a particular burden placed on the most vulnerable—those who have been stereotyped, politically disenfranchised, and excluded from resources that improve their health and social status.

Population health approaches frame health inequities as being structured by the distribution of or access to health-promoting resources that can shape healthier behaviors, increase access to and use of healthcare and social services, and lead to better health outcomes. The disparities that arise at family, community, neighborhood, and other population levels have intersecting determinants. For example, the harms of poverty at the family level might be further amplified by poverty at the neighborhood level (Wickrama et al. 2005).

These determinants require different types of evidence to understand and warrant structural intervention (Umberson and Montez 2010). Therefore, a population health approach can be optimal to address the intersecting social, structural, and political determinants of health, especially when paired with community-engaged strategies (Card et al. 2011; Thomas et al. 2011). Population health approaches can be powerful tools to address contextual, individual, and epigenetic factors that produce poor health outcomes for many communities. We explore population health through the lens of understanding the ongoing impact of racism on the study and practice of public health (Williams et al. 2019; LaVeist 2000). Racism has, in effect, structured power and guided powerbrokers within the academy and the larger public health infrastructure, which includes public health agencies, healthcare, funders, and policymakers. Further, our thinking is driven by an intersectional perspective that also acknowledges the importance of considering other dimensions of oppression, such as structural sexism and classism (Crenshaw 2013; Bowleg 2023).

Structural Racism

The totality of the US infrastructure was built on systems of racism and capitalism (Pirtle 2020; Spector 2014). Both systems have elements of competition, inclusion, and exclusion to create hierarchy; a permanent labor force to support local, national, and multinational interests; and an open or market of ideas that seeks to support and regard private interest as the most dominant. Krieger has defined structural racism at the societal level by characterizing it by the actions societies take to reinforce racial inequities that are reflected in history, interconnected institutions, and culture (Krieger 2014). Bailey and Bassett detail some the specific interconnected institutions, including "...housing, education, employment, earnings, benefits, credit, media, health care, criminal justice, etc) that in turn reinforce discriminatory beliefs, values, and distribution of resources' reflected in history, culture, and interconnected institutions" (Bailey et al. 2017, 1454). These reinforcing systems and structures have produced an industry and culture of racism in the US that accounts for high levels of poverty, racialized residential segregation, stigmatized social and healthcare services, and political disenfranchisement (Michaels et al. 2023). Part of this culture of racism is fortified by White cultural superiority, which seeks to subjugate and repress racial and ethnic minorities (Fanon 1956). The repression of racial and ethnic minorities comes from systemic denial of social mobility opportunities and linking the fate of economic, educational, and health benefits to the many tools and mechanisms of discrimination.

Power, then, becomes formal, systematic, routine, and embedded in informal exchanges between individuals and institutions and in subgoals of corporate interest that can shape a cultural and political environment with a minor focus on equity. Each of these exchanges needs a subsystem to support it, through ideas and/or material resources. This gives rise to the notion of racial capitalism. As Robinson (2021, 2) suggests, "The development, organization, and expansion of capitalist society pursued essentially racial directions, so too did social ideology. As a material force, then, it could be expected that racialism would inevitably permeate the social structures emergent from capitalism ... the term 'racial capitalism' ... refer[s] to this development and to the subsequent structure as a historical agency."

Racial capitalism, for the purpose of this chapter on health, serves as the dominant agent of limited scientific thinking; the systemic denial of racism as a fundamental cause of disease; a small diverse pipeline of scholars, academic institutions that contribute to narratives of White superiority; and how Black health has been sacrificed in pursuit of capitalistic gains. Our fields of science and the processes of scientific inquiry are built upon a history of putting forth theories, models, evidence, and practices that reify the tenets of racial capitalism. Racial capitalism in historical form is exemplified by:

- Chattel slavery, an exploited racialized labor class, which established societal norms for devaluing Black bodies, except to the extent that they advanced the goals of industry and production (Franklin and Moss 2000; Berlin 1998), and the lack of a universal right to healthcare.

- The convict leasing system and its birth of the prison industrial complex using prisons to manufacture goods and to build US infrastructures such as railways (Alexander 2010).
- Tobacco company predatory marketing that targeted campaigns specifically at Black people and in predominantly Black communities, including the Uptown cigarette brand.

Examples of modern racial capitalism include:

- **The Flint Water crisis:** The local government diverted to an unsafe water source that was polluted by local manufacturing. A local plant of a major global manufacturing company avoided using this water source for its own products, while the local community members ingested poor-quality water. Employees were expected to be healthy and productive while consuming unsafe water.
- **Essential workers during the COVID-19 pandemic:** This downgraded the relevance of several occupations and industries to continue working to support the high demand for goods, services, and products, during a public health crisis (Pirtle 2020).
- **The lasting health effects of the sugar industry:** This industry gained strength from chattel slavery, creating an international dependence on sugar, and was a major contributor to chronic diseases within the US food system and to disparities in health (Muhammad 2021).

It is important to explore how racial capitalism gave rise to and was supported by scientific racism. Scientific scholarship has helped to create unchecked dominant narratives about racialized and minoritized groups. Many of these narratives have not had supporting evidence and did not include perspectives or interpretations of evidence by the "subjects" of this research.

Scientific Racism

Scientific racism has been the academic mechanism that justifies and communicates to powerbrokers and leaders of institutions that racialized groups are inferior and should have access only to limited-to-no health and social services and resources that can enhance social mobility. Social scientists during the nineteenth and early twentieth centuries defined Black people—and by extension, other racialized groups—as both biologically and socially inferior (Yudell 2014, Gee et al. 2020). This pseudoscientific belief has prevailed as the primary theory of race yet has been disputed with several lines of evidence. For example, in the same period that Josh Nott characterized Black slaves as a biologically appropriate phenotype for hard labor under trying conditions (1857), Dr. James McCune Smith, the first Black American to earn a medical degree and first Black physician to publish in US medical journals, was using medical science to debunk the idea that racial differences were due to biology (Ioannidis et al. 2021).

Despite dissenting voices and evidence, there were at least three ideologies that promoted scientific racism: social Darwinism, the eugenics movement, and the measurement of intelligence (Dennis 1995; Taylor 1981). This theory of race furthered previous religious and cultural arguments that maintained the institution of slavery and denied the fitness of racialized people to be full citizens in US society or, in other words, suggested that Black and Indigenous people, in particular, were naturally selected to be inferior. These ideas set the foundation for "scientific" studies that set out to buttress the ideology and practice of eugenics (Pernick 1997).

Scientific racism rendered not only Black bodies but all racially minoritized groups invisible in the US by denying that these groups had a history, culture, or skills to make them viable members of the emerging US society post-slavery. W. E. B. Du Bois condemned universities for their participation in this behavior: "The real frontal attack on Reconstruction, as interpreted by the leaders of national thought in 1870 and for some time thereafter, came from the universities and . . . professors of political science and history" (Du Bois, 1935).

These attacks and pseudoscience were promoted by university professors and by professional associations, such as the American Medical Association, the American Sociologist Association, and the American Anthropological Association.

Historic examples of scientific racism include:

- The 1851 description of drapetomania as a disease of enslaved persons who run away. Those who escaped were believed to have smaller brains and blood vessels, leading to their indolence (Opara et al. 2022).
- The 1932 US Public Health Service Tuskegee Untreated Syphilis Study, previously referred to as the Tuskegee Study of Untreated Syphilis in the Negro Male. This study enrolled over 600 men with and without syphilis without informed consent and told them they were being treated for "bad blood" in exchange for free healthcare exams, meals, and burial insurance (White 2000).

- Doctors unethically took samples of cancer cells from Henrietta Lacks in 1951 while treating her. Researchers learned that her cells were able to survive and reproduce under many laboratory conditions. Her cells were shared widely and became part of the biological research canon under the name HeLa (Sloot 2017).

Contemporary examples of scientific racism include:

- The 1965 Moynihan Report, which described Black families as being in decline and deep peril. This report fueled conservative policies (Moynahan 2011).
- The first targeted marketing of BiDil, a congestive heart failure drug, to Black Americans explicitly. This supports the biological basis of race and promotes a racialized genetic/personalized medicine (Garrod 2006; Kahn 2008). Meanwhile, the real reason BiDil was promoted only for Black patients was because the clinical trials for BiDil only included Black patients, therefore introducing and reflecting racist ideologies into the scientific process.
- In March 2020, the US President referred to COVID-19 as the "Chinese virus," inflaming anti-Asian hate and violence toward Asian American communities (Hswen et al. 2021).

Because of these examples and others, 2020 saw an unprecedented embrace of racism as a public health crisis, acknowledgments of systemic and structural racism, apologies for institutional participation in structural racism, professional associations reconciling for their promotion of biological-race practices and practices performed without consent, recognition of the systemic denial of rights and services withheld from racialized communities in the US, and public statements about and verbal acknowledgments of the unlawful seizure and removal of Indigenous people across the US. For example, the National Institutes of Health created the UNITE initiative to combat structural racism, and the American Medical Association created guidelines to address structural racism (American Medical Association 2021; Bernard et al. 2022; National Institutes of Health n.d.). Just years before, the study of racism was deemed too political and biased, so these efforts are signs of progress. We still do not largely acknowledge descendants of Africans enslaved in the US as a distinct group that needs intervention (Dean and Smith 2021). However, while a public shift has occurred toward thinking about racism, a shift in practice has largely not occurred. We offer up a shift in frameworks, theories, and models to further guide the attention toward antiracist public health practices to achieve equity in health at the population level.

How Theories Around Health are Limited by Scientific Racism

Just as race theory molded biological-race thinking and analysis, so has a focus in public health on individual-level theories and models that seek to explain behavior change. Public health research and interventions have depended on individual behavior change without a clear focus on either developing, implementing, or generating evidence about the role of theories and interventions emerging from other disciplines, that can address social and physical environments (Monolo-Pedro et al. 2023). One major issue is that many existing theories focus on individual outcomes, but such approaches are inherently inadequate in explaining group-level outcomes (i.e., racial inequities).

This does not suggest that there are no theories and models that address social and physical environments. This is a call to action for more, a call to integrate them into our public health training, and a call for these models to guide the direction of funders' resources to enhance their strategies on higher levels of the social ecological model and for models that can address structural and social issues that negatively shape health outcomes and constrain health behaviors (Mannor and Malcoe 2022). Much of the evidence around structural racism and health has been limited. The legacy of these studies has generated evidence from studying psychosocial associations of racism and stress through biological, interpersonal, carceral, and institutional pathways; self-reports of discrimination (everyday, cumulative, and from social environments); and state-level structural racism through measures of political participation, employment and job status, educational attainment, and judicial treatment (Bailey et al. 2017; Ford et al. 2019; Gee and Ford 2011). Evidence has been limited because of our scientific approaches and the industry of science production, which has denied the advancement of research, measurement, and interventions around structural mechanisms of racism and health (Thomas et al. 2011; Williams et al. 2019; Ford et al. 2019; Shaw-Ridley and Ridley 2010).

Example: Social Capital, Social Mobility, and Disparities in Health

The concept of social capital grows from the observation that social relationships can create a form of capital that can have effects on multiple outcomes, including health (McKenzie et al. 2002; Harpham et al. 2002; Harpham 2008).

Bourdieu's 1986 concept of social capital addresses issues of resources and access. The Putnam model of social capital does not directly address the relevance of (1) actual or potential resources that are uniquely housed within social networks that may be used for personal or collective action or (2) power dynamics and how people access, or may be denied access to, network-based resources (Wakefield and Poland 2005; Carpiano 2008). Instead, most indicators of social capital are focused on horizontal relationships between friends, family, neighbors, or community members and less on the vertical relationships between individuals, communities, neighborhoods, organizations and sources of power, and decision makers (Kawachi et al. 1997).

These definitions and indicators of social capital may not fully resonate with the daily interactions between individuals within a given community or neighborhood. Results from a case study in the Bushwick neighborhood of Brooklyn, New York, showed that for residents in that area, "trust among neighbors" was not the central factor that mattered for health. There was conflict that reflected the community's widespread distrust toward institutions of power (e.g., the police). Community members expressed this distrust publicly. These higher levels of distrust were the informal strategies residents used to express their concerns, develop social norms, and challenge decision-makers to address issues of crime and the lack of opportunity. Community members felt free to express themselves and were empowered by these opportunities to change their social conditions (Friedman et al. 2007).

This example highlights the limitations of theories and measurement of social interactions based on the current views of how theories operate. Most public health theories suggest that behaviors are made from a rational choice perspective and that individuals have full control. These theories can largely ignore behaviors that may not be viewed as rational or logical. This Brooklyn community found a sense of community from being actively engaged in conflict awareness and resolutions. Their strategies for problem-solving reflect a social reality that is not predictable, which is counter to how theories are utilized in research and interventions. This example also highlights the role of strengths within communities to address disparate health conditions that are not readily observed without in-depth and community-led research strategies (Gilbert et al. 2022; Gilbert et al. 2018).

Other work has suggested that because of oppressive forces that limit expression of forms of social capital (e.g., voter suppression) (Gilbert et al. 2022; Dean and Gilbert 2010), certain groups may need unique indicators of social capital. For example, block parties or street festivals have been found to be a unique form of social capital for Black communities and may be opportunities for health promotion for Black communities (Dean 2015). An explicit attention to racism could expand social capital theory's usefulness for understanding health and racial health inequities.

Example: Theory of Gender and Power as a Template for Centering Those Who Are Othered

We can learn from theories that connect power, labor, and the social, economic, and health risks women experience to racial and scientific racism. Wingood and DiClemente (2000) use Connell's theory of gender and power to explain women's risk to HIV exposure:

> "One consequence of "otherizing" women is that they become defined in terms of their similarity and dissimilarity to men. Another consequence of otherizing women is that they become defined in terms of their functional significance to men rather than in terms of their own significance." (539–540)

> "An elaboration of the theory of gender and power proposes that the three social structures (the structures of labor, power, and cathexis) exist at the societal and institutional levels and are maintained in institutions by social mechanisms. The social mechanisms produce gender-based inequities and disparities (e.g. in women's economic potential, women's control of resources, and gender-based expectations of women's role in society). These inequities and disparities are apparent in the public health, social and behavioral sciences, and medical fields as exposures, risk factors, and biological properties. These exposures, risk factors, and biological properties all interact to increase women's vulnerability to diseases, including HIV." (541)

In their application of Connell's theory, these authors have helped to explain how women can become vulnerable because of their social position, limits to their access because of their gender identity, stigma and stereotypes assigned to women, and other forms of gender-based subjugation (Connell 1987). Their power, either perceived or real, is gender-based. This theory suggests that men and other women communicate about the needs, resources, and opportunities for women as framed by viewing women in comparison to men. The application of this theory provides an opportunity to develop studies and interventions from an introspective view of women. This means that, without a clear understanding of a woman's-world view and individual and collective experiences, any public health approach will be limited and not sustainable. The social norms constructed about women should become integral to research, interventions, and public health practices to advance a population-health approach. Similarly, in seeking to develop public health interventions that promote racial health equity, we must center the experiences of racial and ethnic minorities, as opposed to only viewing them in contrast to White populations.

Conclusion

We have outlined a description of racial capitalism and scientific racism and how they shape population health outcomes. Without an understanding of these structural and institutional forms of racism, our scholarship will continue to be limited and our interventions, impotent. Population health requires a unique analysis of risk, assets, and opportunity. These are not necessarily the language of forms of racism that only seek to "otherize" populations through structural and institutional mechanisms. It is our charge to upend these practices within the academy to ensure that our social science theories and methodology reflect the lived experiences of the most vulnerable. We cannot rely solely on current social science methods, because of their traditional focus on individuals rather than communities or structures. Many of these methods are colorblind and ignore the various forms of racism. This reifies both racial capitalism and scientific racism and objectifies racialized communities. Ignoring these issues ensures that efforts working toward health equity will only be ones of words without deeds.

References

Alexander, Michelle. 2010. *The New Jim Crow: Mass Incarceration in the Age of Colorblindness.* New York: New Press.

American Medical Association. 2021. "AMA Adopts Guidelines That Confront Systemic Racism in Medicine." https://www.ama-assn.org/press-center/press-releases/ama-adopts-guidelines-confront-systemic-racism-medicine.

Bailey, Zinzi D., Nancy Krieger, Madina Agénor, and Jasmine Graves. 2017. "Structural Racism and Health Inequities in the USA: Evidence and Interventions." *Lancet* 389 (10077): 1453–1463.

Berlin, Ira. 1998. *Many Thousands Gone: The First Two Centuries of Slavery in North America.* Cambridge, MA: Harvard University Press.

Bernard, Marie A., Alfred C. Johnson, and Tara A. Schwetz. 2022. "UNITE Progress Report: 2021-2022." https://www.nih.gov/sites/default/files/research-training/initiatives/ending-structural-racism/UNITE-progress-report-2022.pdf

Bourdieu, Pierre. 2011. "The forms of capital (1986)." *Cultural theory: An anthology* 1 (81-93): 949.

Bowleg, L. 2023. "Beyond Intersectional Identities: Ten Intersectional Structural Competencies for Critical Health Equity Research." In *Routledge Companion to Intersectionalities*, edited by Nash, Jennifer C., and Samantha Pinto, 101–116. Routledge.

Card, Josefina J., Julie Solomon, and Shayna D. Cunningham. 2011. "How to Adapt Effective Programs for Use in New Contexts." *Health Promotion Practice* 12 (1): 25–35.

Carpiano, R. M. 2008. "Actual or potential neighborhood resources and access to them: Testing hypotheses of social capital for the health of female caregivers". *Social science & medicine* 67 (4), 568–582.

Connell, R. W. 1987. *Gender and Power*. Stanford, CA: Stanford University Press.

Crenshaw, K. W. 2013. "Mapping the Margins: Intersectionality, Identity Politics, and Violence against Women of Color." In *In The Public Nature of Private Violence*, edited by Martha Fineman and Roxanne Mykitiuk, 93–118. Routledge.

Dean, Lorraine, and Keon L. Gilbert. 2010. "Social Capital and Political Advocacy for African American Health." *Harvard Journal of African American Public Policy* 16: 85.

Dean, L. T., A. Hillier, H. Chau-Glendinning, S. Subramanian, D. R., Williams, & I. Kawachi. 2015. "Can you party your way to better health? A propensity score analysis of block parties and health." *Social Science & Medicine* 138: 201–209.

Dean, Lorraine T., and Genee S. Smith. 2021. "Examining the Role of Family History of US Enslavement in Health Care System Distrust Today." *Ethnicity & Disease* 31 (3): 417.

Dennis, Rutledge M. 1995. "Social Darwinism, Scientific Racism, and the Metaphysics of Race." *Journal of Negro Education* 64 (3): 243–252.

Du Bois, W.E. Burghardt. 1935. "Black Reconstruction." *An Essay Toward a History of the Part which Black Folk Played in the Attempt to Reconstruct Democracy in America, 1860-1880*, 718–720.

Fanon, F. 1956. "Racism and Culture." Frantz Fanon's speech before the First Congress of Negro Writers and Artists in Paris, September 1956. Published in the Special Issue of Presence Africaine, June-November, 1956.

Ford, Chandra L., Derek M. Griffith, Marino A. Bruce, and Keon L. Gilbert, eds. 2019. *Racism: Science and Tools for the Public Health Professional*. Washington, DC: American Public Health Association.

Franklin, John Hope, and E. Higginbotham. 2024. *From Slavery to Freedom: A History of African Americans, 10th edition*. McGraw Hill: New York.

Friedman, Samuel R., Pedro Mateu-Gelabert, R. Curtis, Carey Maslow, Melissa Bolyard, Milagros Sandoval, Peter L. Flom. 2007. "Social Capital or Networks,

Negotiations, and Norms? A Neighborhood Case Study." *American Journal of Preventive Medicine* 32 (6: S160–S170.

Garrod, Joel Z. 2006. "A Brave Old World: An Analysis of Scientific Racism and BiDil." *McGill Journal of Medicine* 9 (1): 54–60.

Gee, G. C., M. J. Ro, A. W. Rimoin. 2020. "Seven Reasons to Care about Racism and COVID-19 and Seven Things to Do to Stop It." *American Journal of Public Health* 110 (7: 954–955.

Gee, Gilbert C., and Chandra L. Ford. 2011. "Structural Racism and Health Inequities: Old Issues, New Directions." *Du Bois Review* 8 (1): 115–132.

Gilbert, Keon L., Stephanie M. McClure, and Mary Shaw-Ridley. 2018. "Changing Health Outcomes through Community-Driven Processes: Implications for Practice and Research." In *Public Health Research Methods for Partnerships and Practice*, edited by Melody S. Goodman and Vetta Sanders Thompson, 301–315. New York: CRC Press.

Gilbert, Keon L., Yusuf Ransome, Lorraine T. Dean, Jerell DeCaille, and I. Kawachi. 2022. "Social Capital, Black Social Mobility, and Health Disparities." *Annual Review of Public Health* 43: 173–191.

Harpham, T., Grant, E., & Thomas, E. 2002. "Measuring social capital within health surveys: key issues." *Health policy and planning*, 17(1), 106–111.

Harpham, T. 2008. "The measurement of community social capital through surveys." In *Social Capital and Health*, edited by I Kawachi, SV Subramanian, D Kim, 51–62. New York: Springer Science + Business Media LLC.

Hswen, Y., X. Xu, A. Hing, J. B. Hawkins, J. S. Brownstein, and G. C. Gee.2021. "Association of '# Covid19' versus '# Chinesevirus' with Anti-Asian Sentiments on Twitter: March 9–23, 2020." *American Journal of Public Health* 111 (5): 956–964.

Ioannidis, John P.A., Neil R. Powe, and Clyde Yancy. 2021. "Recalibrating the Use of Race in Medical Research." *JAMA* 325 (7): 623–624.

Kahn, Jonathan. 2008. "Beyond Bidil: The Expanding Embrace of Race in Biomedical Research and Product Development." *Saint Louis University Journal of Health Law & Policy* 86: 61–92.

Kawachi, I., B. P. Kennedy, K. Lochner, & D. Prothrow-Stith. 1997. "Social capital, income inequality, and mortality." *American journal of public health* 87 (9), 1491–1498.

Krieger, Nancy. 2014. "Discrimination and Health Inequities." *International Journal of Health Services* 44 (4): 643–710.

LaVeist, Thomas A. 2000. "On the Study of Race, Racism, and Health: A Shift from Description to Explanation." *International Journal of Health Services* 30 (1): 217–219.

Manalo-Pedro, E., Walsemann, K. M., and Gee, G. C. 2023. "Whose Knowledge Heals? Transforming Teaching in the Struggle for Health Equity." *Health Education & Behavior* 50 (4): 482–492.

Mannor, K. M., and L. H. Malcoe. 2022. "Uses of Theory in Racial Health Disparities Research: A Scoping Review and Application of Public Health Critical Race Praxis." *Annals of Epidemiology* 66: 56–64.

McKenzie, K., R. Whitley, & S. Weich (2002). "Social capital and mental health." *The British Journal of Psychiatry* 181 (4), 280–283.

Michaels, E. K., T. Lam-Hine, T. T. Nguyen, G. C. Gee, and A. M. Allen. 2023. "The Water Surrounding the Iceberg: Cultural Racism and Health Inequities." *Milbank Quarterly* 101 (3): 768–814.

Muhammad, Khalil Gibran. 2021. "Sugar." In *The 1619 Project: A New Origin Story*, edited by and Jake Silverstein, Nikole Hannah-Jones, Caitlin Roper, and Ilena Silverman, 71–87. New York: One World.

"National Institutes of Health," n.d. "Ending Structural Racism: UNITE." https://www.nih.gov/ending-structural-racism/unite.

Obama, Barack. 2008. "A More Perfect Union." https://www.youtube.com/watch?v=pWe7wTVbLUU.

Opara, Ijeoma Nnodim, Latonya Riddle-Jones, and Nakia Allen. 2022. "Modern Day Drapetomania: Calling Out Scientific Racism." *Journal of General Internal Medicine* 37 (1): 225–225.

Pernick, M. S. 1997. "Eugenics and Public Health in American History." *American Journal of Public Health* 87 (11): 1767–1772.

Pirtle, Whitney N. Laster. 2020. "Racial Capitalism: A Fundamental Cause of Novel Coronavirus (COVID-19) Pandemic Inequities in the United States." *Health Education Behavior* 47 (4): 504–508.

Robinson, Cedric J. 2021. *Black Marxism: The Making of the Black Radical Tradition*. Revised and updated 3rd ed. Chapel Hill: University of North Carolina Press.

Shaw-Ridley, Mary, and Charles R. Ridley. 2010. "The Health Disparities Industry: Is It an Ethical Conundrum?" *Health Promotion Practice* 11 (4): 454–464.

Sloot, Rebecca. 2017. *The Immortal Life of Henrietta Lacks*. Broadway Books.

Spector, A. 2014. "Racism and Capitalism—Crisis and Resistance: Exploring the Dynamic between Class Oppression and Racial Oppression." *Humanity & Society* 38 (2): 116–131.

Taylor, Carol M. 1981. "W.E.B. DuBois's Challenge to Scientific Racism." *Journal of Black Studies* 11 (4): 449–460.

Thomas, Stephen B., Sandra Crouse Quinn, James Butler, Craig S. Fryer, and Mary A. Garza. 2011. "Toward a Fourth Generation of Disparities Research to Achieve Health Equity." *Annual Review of Public Health* 32: 399–416.

Umberson, Debra, and Jennifer Karas J. K. Montez. 2010. "Social Relationships and Health: A Flashpoint for Health Policy." *Journal of Health and Social Behavior* 51: 1–16.

U.S. Department of Labor, Office of Policy Planning and Research. 1965. The Negro Family: The Case for National Action. Washington, DC: U.S. Department of Labor. http://www.dol.gov/oasam/programs/history/webidmeynihan.htm.

Wakefield, S. E. L, B. Poland. 2005. "Family, friend or foe? Critical reflections on the relevance and role of social capital in health promotion and community development." *Social Science & Medicine.* 60 (12): 2819–2832.

White, Robert M. 2000. "Unraveling the Tuskegee Study of Untreated Syphilis." *Archives of Internal Medicine* 160 (5): 585–598.

Wickrama, K. A. S., Samuel Noh, and Chalandra M. Bryant. 2005. "Racial Differences in Adolescent Distress: Differential Effects of the Family and Community for Blacks and Whites." *Journal of Community Psychology* 33 (3): 261–282.

Williams, David R., Jourdyn A. Lawrence, and Brigette A. Davis. 2019. "Racism and Health: Evidence and Needed Research." *Annual Review of Public Health* 40: 105–125.

Wingood, Gina M., and Ralph J. DiClemente. 2000. "Application of the Theory of Gender and Power to Examine HIV-Related Exposures, Risk Factors, and Effective Interventions for Women." *Health Education & Behavior* 27 (5): 539–565.

Yudell, M. 2014. *Race Unmasked: Biology and Race in the Twentieth Century*. New York: Columbia University Press.

Chapter 9

Orienting Public Health Pedagogy: Using Anti-oppression Tools for Teaching Privilege and Health

Keilah Jacques, anushka aqil, Krystal Lee, and Graham Mooney

Introduction

The field of public health is at a critical juncture in relation to systemic oppression and its impact on health and well-being. Organizations ranging from school districts to city governments to professional organizations coalesce around the phrases "systemic oppression negatively impacts health" and "racism is a public health crisis" (Mock 2020). Drs. Jennifer Garcia and Meinah Sharif (2015) offer a call to action for public health educators, practitioners, and researchers, noting that "public health, at its core, is antiracist work." Yet very little training exists to orient and guide public health teachers, researchers, and practitioners toward the individual and institutional transformations needed to forge a genuine reorientation away from systemic oppression. North American health education faculty often avoid having conversations around oppressive systems like racism, sexism, trans/homophobia, and casteism because they feel unprepared to do so (aqil 2021). This results in a cycle of unprepared public health practitioners who struggle to recognize oppressive ideologies like White Supremacy Culture (WSC or white supremacy) and their associated systems of oppression that affect public health at the level of the social determinants of health (SDoH). When unaware of these systems of oppression, not only do public health practitioners further reinforce negative stereotypes and ideologies, but health practitioners, researchers, and teachers are ill-prepared to critically examine the contextual systems of the SDoH and orient away from them. We can take advantage of the current prevailing mood in favor of addressing systemic oppression by training public health

Keilah Jacques et al., *Orienting Public Health Pedagogy: Using Anti-oppression Tools for Teaching Privilege and Health.* In: *Power, Privilege, and Public Health in the United States.* Edited by: Lorraine T. Dean and Keilah A. Jacques, Oxford University Press. © Oxford University Press (2025). DOI: 10.1093/9780197760956.003.0009 practitioners to improve their awareness of these systems and equipping them with tools to dismantle them. To accomplish this, public health education has the opportunity and responsibility to examine current pedagogical approaches and redesign courses in alignment with anti-oppressive principles.

This chapter offers guidance for public health educators seeking to dismantle oppressive systems in policy, practice, and research by first learning about the ideology of WSC and how the characteristics associated with power and privilege show up in our learning environments. We then discuss the principles of anti-oppression and offer pedagogical and curricular examples of how current and future faculty can make this shift in their classrooms. As a result of offering insight into the crux of oppressive systems and then distinguishing a method designed to orient away from these systems, we hope to pinpoint tools that allow educators and learners to exemplify anti-oppressive and antiracist public health practice.

Systems and Ideologies of Oppression

An ideology is a way of thinking that is central to the development of beliefs and practices, in both personal identity and the way society holds itself together (Nescolarde-Selva et al. 2017). The characteristics of ideologies include but are not limited to: the process of production of meaning, signs (iconography), and value in society; a body of ideal characteristics of a particular social group or class; and ideas that help to legitimate a dominant political power (Kishimoto 2018). Each of these elements can be found in the dominant pedagogical approaches of higher education, including public health. This point is illustrated in the seminal work, *The Hidden Curriculum and Moral Education* by Henry Giroux (1983). Giroux argues that power is intimately tied to ideology and that schools play a crucial role in reproducing dominant ideologies. He contends that schools are not neutral institutions but are shaped by the social and economic forces that surround them—in particular, forces that function to perpetuate and uphold systemic oppression at the expense of the marginalized for the benefit of the power-holding elite. Examining ideologies means examining the dominant ideas, meanings, and values found not only in social and cultural influences but also in pedagogy—as education occupies the role of power brokering.

The term *system of oppression* describes the hierarchical and intersecting societal, social, economic, and political norms and practices that systematically disadvantaged groups in ways that are interconnected and mutually reinforcing, based on identity (e.g., religion, race, sexual orientation) and circumstance (e.g., socioeconomic status, ability) and lead some members of society to a dehumanization and disconnection from accessing well-being, opportunity, quality of life, and dignity (Collins 2000; Crenshaw 1989; Lorde 1984).

Systems of oppression are maintained by ideologies and show up in functional form as policies, practices, and procedures. Ideologies of White superiority also drive systems of oppression that are common in higher education. White Supremacy Culture (WSC) is one such ideology that pervades and perpetuates oppressive systems. White supremacy refers to the ways in which the pseudoscientific concepts of race and whiteness are used to establish a "hierarchy of racialized value" (Collins 2000; Crenshaw 1989; Lorde 1984). Consequently, WSC reflects the norms, beliefs, and standards of whiteness as ideal, resulting in overt and covert valuing of whiteness and devaluing of nonwhiteness, with a particular bent toward anti-Blackness (Okun 2021). This ideology perpetuates often-unnamed, unseen cultural norms. Such norms are used to broker power that maintains vast and violent structures of inequity (Johnson and Joseph-Salisbury 2018; Okun 2021) WSC teaches us, for example, that Blackness is valueless, dangerous, and threatening and that Indigenous communities no longer exist outside of exoticized, romanticized, and culturally appropriated stereotypes. This ideology "pits other races and racial groups against each other while always defining them as inferior to the white group" (Okun 2021). This results in laws, policies, procedures, and practices that reflect a culture committed to prioritizing profit over treating people, especially people of color, humanely and with dignity.

Another oppressive ideology that shows up in classrooms is intellectual domination, which imposes neoliberal, Western, and White supremacist values on the process of knowledge creation. These values are promoted when instructors serve as agents of WSC and transmit dominant ideas in pedagogies and curricula (Allen 2015; hooks 1994). In this way, anyone of any race can perpetuate WSC. Though there has been some scholarly examination of ideological influence in public health education, and there is emergent literature on instructor training, studies that concentrate on oppressive ideologies are scant, or dated (aqil et al. 2021). Without a critical examination of oppressive ideologies, and the cultural elements active in themselves, educators may disengage from conversations about, for example, racism in the classroom or, further, may rely on their understanding of racialized differences, which in many cases reflects dominant ideals and views. Educators' tools and training are needed to understand the role of education in maintaining racial hegemony, a focus that is beyond the scope of this chapter.

Several renowned critical scholars have argued that higher education institutions are simultaneously sites of oppression and emancipation (Collins 2000; hooks 1994; Mohanty 2014). Critical instructors demonstrate agency when they resist traditional learning and utilize the classroom as a democratic space for collective interrogation of the nature of knowledge, power, racism, class, corporate systems, policy, media, and other sociocultural issues that contextualize the social determinants of health (hooks 1994). Evidence suggests that even a single class can change learners' perspectives on the role of privilege and power in health professional practice and can cause questioning of dominant socialization patterns (Witten and Maskarinec 2015).

White Supremacy Culture (WSC) Ideology, Power, and Privilege

In 2021, Okun defined the concept of White Supremacy Culture (WSC), thus naming and acknowledging the cultural norms used to broker power and maintain vast and violent structures of inequity (Okun 2021; Johnson and Joseph-Salisbury 2018). Okun (2021) identifies thirteen characteristics of WSC, which stem from the political and social organizing ideology of white superiority. Though the list consists of thirteen characteristics, this paper will focus on five that are often present in higher education pedagogical and curricular norms.

These five characteristics highlight power as a central component of ideological implementation and intellectual domination. They are worship of the written word, power hoarding, the right to comfort, paternalism, and objectivity.

Worship of the written word is defined as honoring only what is written to a narrow standard (Okun 2021). This includes an erasure of the wide range of ways we communicate with each other and leads to disconnection. Worship of the written word can manifest in pedagogy as a focus on information sharing that is restricted to formally recognized methodologies of teaching. These methodologies often center on dominant hegemonic ideas expressed in objective forms and verified solely by empirical evidence. Often this means an ironclad syllabus, utilization of only peer-reviewed texts, and text-heavy content delivery, which themselves indicate the significance of gatekeeping by the editors and reviewers of scholarly journals. Additionally, learning is qualified by written skill, strong documentation of completion, and "original" work referenced by White-dominant, Western-centric, academic thought.

Power hoarding is defined as little, if any, value in sharing power. Because power is seen as limited, those with power feel threatened when anyone suggests changes in how things should be done. Moreover, they feel that suggestions for change reflect their leadership (Okun 2021). In pedagogy, this characteristic is demonstrated through teaching that focuses on rote memorization and regurgitation of ideas, methodologies, and perspectives. This "teaching to the test" is usually didactic, focuses primarily on examinations, and is concerned with knowledge demonstration at the lowest level of Bloom's taxonomy.[1] In course design, a didactic-only teaching style leaves no room for collaborative learning activities, voices of marginalized populations, or critical praxis as a means to demonstrate learning.

The right to comfort is defined as the belief that those with power have a right to emotional and psychological comfort. This often results in scapegoating those who cause discomfort, equating individual acts of unfairness against White people with systemic racism that targets people of color (Okun 2021. In the classroom, this can be seen through disassociating the personal and political role of teaching (hooks 1994). Much like power hoarding, this characteristic leaves no room in the teaching process to engage in critical practices such as presenting alternate views or interrogating systems. In curriculum design, it is personified by instructors who discuss tangentially or omit completely any examination of racism, racialized systems, racist ideologies, or other forms of oppression.

Paternalism is characterized by those with power assuming they are capable of making decisions for and in the interests of those without power, assuming it is not important or necessary to understand the viewpoint or experience of those for whom they are making decisions (Okun, 2021). In pedagogy, this characteristic manifests itself through the maintenance of hierarchical power structures, where faculty are intellectually dominant and utilize source material that perpetuates the dominant worldview. Paternalism is present when instructors engage in the banking model, which presumes the instruction is all-knowing and is the only form of authoritative knowledge, versus collaborative learning from diverse authors, community members, and students (Freire 2000; hooks 1994). Similarly, it is present in generalizations about data

---

[1] "The Taxonomy of Educational Objectives, commonly referred to as Bloom's taxonomy, was originally published in 1956 to inform and standardize assessments of educational achievement, and describes a hierarchy of cognitive processes (Bloom, 1956). Bloom's taxonomy is in effect a theory of how students learn, with mastery of lower-level cognitive skills required before higher-order skills can be obtained" (Callaghan-Koru and Aqil 2022).

or populations without examining the context and power structure related to the examples or case studies provided.

Objectivity is defined by the belief that emotions are inherently destructive and irrational and should not play a role in decision-making or group processes. It requires people to think linearly and ignores or invalidates those who think in other ways (Okun 2021). Pedagogically, this practice can be found when critical reflection is excluded as a teaching tool and students are not encouraged to participate in subjective meaning-making that incorporates their identities, lived experiences, or perspectives. In curriculum design, instructors practice objectivity when discussion, practicum opportunities, and capstones exclude positional evaluations and meaning-making through dialectic activities or reflective praxis.

Dismantling WSC in the classroom requires the application of educational frameworks and teaching approaches that examine the ideologies of dominance and subordination within the social agreements (ways we agree to be together, ways we agree to function inside intuitions and systems, and so on) of public health policy, practice, and research. The essential feature of achieving health equity lies in the ability to deconstruct the structural barriers and apply new principles of practice in health-related opportunities, resources, and experiences.

Shifting to an Anti-oppressive Ideology

Anti-oppressive ideology is grounded in the "eradication of oppression through institutional and structural changes" (Sakamoto and Pitner 2005). This requires an awareness "that society is not based on equal distribution of power and privilege and that sociopolitical and economic discourses maintain a division between the privileged and the disadvantaged" (McDonald 2008).

Anti-oppression is informed by several theories and frameworks that include postmodernism, Black thought, antiracism, Indigenous thought, queer theory, anticolonialism, feminism, and intersectionality theory (Campbell 2003; Dalrymple and Burke 2006). It seeks to recognize and challenge power imbalances (Strier and Binyamin 2014) that shape how individuals, communities, and systems operate; it is both a theory and a practice-based approach aimed at advancing social justice and equity (Yee et al. 2015). Anti-oppression centers critical self-reflection and acknowledgment of power, privilege, and politics and prioritizes effecting change at both the micro- and macrolevels (Dalrymple and Burke 2006). As such, anti-oppression focuses on training practitioners to be cognizant of their own roles and the context within which they are working to address complicated public health issues.

Anti-oppressive action commonly involves unlearning one's previous (mis-)understanding of how power operates in society and relearning a more coherent intersectional analysis. A critical and self-reflexive lens is a crucial component of anti-oppressive practice in order to identify one's own relationship to upholding systems of oppression—especially when one is in a position of privilege (Kumashiro 2000; Lavallée 2014).

Within education, anti-oppression is seen as a process—a framework that is ever-evolving and shifting as new knowledge is acquired, power dynamics shift, and definitions change. This implies that there is a need for continuing professional education in anti-oppression that spans an educator's lifetime (Kumashiro 2000). More specifically, anti-oppression provides five principles through which to engage in anti-oppressive practice:

1. **Context:** We must acknowledge that the actions and behaviors of individuals and organizations are contextualized within a historical and geographical conditions.
2. **Power:** We must acknowledge that relations differ and are complex across individual and organizational levels; as such, they need to be analyzed according to who has power and how fruits of that power are accessed or denied.
3. **The personal and the political are linked:** We must acknowledge that individuals are situated within a broader social context and their life is viewed and experienced in relation to multiple social systems.
4. **Social differences:** We must acknowledge that power relations are influenced by social differences and therefore impact experiences of oppression and privilege.
5. **Critical self-reflection:** Individuals need to be cognizant of their identities and the impact of personal experiences and be aware of the wider contexts that affect us indirectly or directly (Clifford 1995).

When applied to course content and teaching methodologies, anti-oppressive principles provide specific steps that instructors can take to examine their teaching methods and curriculum design. They offer a guide for educators to engage with issues of history (context), structural bias, and power and can be applied in conjunction with other frameworks relevant to the course content or area of expertise. Incorporating anti-oppressive principles into public health curricula offers a prime opportunity to prepare future public health practitioners to address the needs of the field and challenge systems of oppression.

Challenges to Shifting Ideology

While many educators value and acknowledge the importance of discussing equity issues in the classroom, they admit to not feeling equipped or comfortable teaching this content from an informed lens (Aslop 2018; Brownell and Tanner 2012; Kim and Del Prado 2019; Koblinsky and Clark 2015). Our experience and that of others (Lyons et al. 2023) working to shift ideology and transform pedagogy is that there are many challenges and obstacles, from the amount of time it takes to train teachers to competing institutional priorities, the lack of resources for pedagogy, and discomfort on the part of faculty (Chávez et al. 2006; Leonardo and Porter 2010).

Manalo-Pedro et al. write, "Unlearning oppressive ideologies may feel strange and unsettling, given the myriad of societal norms which elevate educators above students, naturalize racial hierarchies, and depoliticize death" (Manalo-Pedro et al. 2023, 487). However, as yet, no blueprint exists on how public health institutions can reorient toward anti-oppression (Chandler 2022). Departmental and institutional support is an important facilitator of anti-oppression practices in pedagogy (Lyons et al. 2023), as it commits resources and provides a form of legitimacy (Polston et al. 2023). An example of committing resources is to train faculty in how to deliver anti-oppression pedagogy (Kalbarczyk et al. 2023); while it is possible to implement anti-oppression principles at the classroom level regardless of institutional support, it is less contentious and holistic if there is organizational commitment (Lyons et al. 2023). When implementing anti-oppressive principles in a course on injuries and violence in an epidemiology department, Lyons et al. found that the "generous grading policies"—such as credit/no credit assignments, no late penalties—were well received by many students, but a few preferred a "higher standard for grading" (Lyons et al. 2023). Thinking of such grading policies as "generous," on the one hand, and of a lower standard, on the other, indicates an unwillingness to relinquish the punitive norms of grading structures that perpetuate WSC.

Shifting Curriculum Design and Pedagogy

Freire identifies the banking model of education as a concept that reflects an imbalance of power in the classroom, with instructors holding all the power (i.e., knowledge) and the students holding none. This pedagogical approach serves as a model of hierarchy, dominance, and oppressive power structures that students then play out in life. As an alternative, Freire

(2000) promotes education as the practice of freedom that must be modeled by the instructor *and* taught in the curriculum—knowledge and critical pedagogy.

Critical pedagogy is anchored in the belief that educators should equip students to build the skill in, and model for learners, the practice of examining power, structures, and inequitable patterns within systems and structures. Critical pedagogy sees education as fundamentally political because it is rooted in a liberatory and revolutionary struggle to subvert and dismantle oppression in various forms. For Freire (2000), this is education as the practice of freedom. To shift the practice of teaching toward anti-oppression, educators must prioritize collectivist forms of learning that are based in critical thinking and principled action rather than hegemonic ideas of dominance and hierarchical uses of power. Next, we offer examples of how to shift course design and evaluation to reflect anti-oppressive principles.

Examples and Recommendations

Worship of the Written Word

The written word is a "form of knowing" (Freire 2000). Course syllabi, assignments, and examinations tend to be dominated by resources that are text-centered and therefore privilege White, Western, global north methods of knowledge communication. In particular, they ignore equally valuable oral and visual forms of communication that are central to other knowledge traditions. There are many ways that curricular components can orient away from the worship of the written word. For example, syllabi can include podcasts and videos reflecting a range of viewpoints that come from inside and outside the academy. In-class discussions can draw on the collective knowledge of students themselves and incorporate the lived experiences of community partners (if an authentic relationship exists with community partners). Assignments and final exams need not be in written format to demonstrate competency. There are a variety of examples of how to design "un-essays," ranging from podcasting to engagement on social media (Irwin 2022). Many students appreciate the opportunity to engage with nonwritten formats particularly when rubrics and evaluation criteria are clear. It is important to stress that learners will need appropriate and robust scaffolding in how to make choices about their own learning, practice active listening, analyze nonwritten material, produce audio-visual media like a podcast or video, create effective visual content, and so on. This may require the teacher to acknowledge the limits of their own pedagogical training, and the additional resources needed for this may present a barrier to implementation.

It is not lost on the authors that the field needs systematic evaluation to identify competency for practice, which can be challenging if students are submitting different types of products. However, one way to address this may be for the field to move toward competency-based learning, standardizing demonstrable skills, and incorporating rubrics that are based on types of demonstrable practices. This is the current road the field of nursing is taking as a result of the American Association of Colleges of Nursing (AACN) establishing "The Essentials." The AACN works to establish accreditation and quality standards for nursing education; assists schools in implementing those standards; influences the nursing profession to improve healthcare; and promotes public support for professional nursing education, research, and practice (American Association of Colleges of Nursing n.d.). The Essentials define quality in nursing education and outline the necessary curriculum content and expected competencies of graduates from baccalaureate, master's, and doctor of nursing practice programs (American Association of Colleges of Nursing n.d.).

Power Hoarding

Anti-oppressive practice approaches power hoarding by diffusing power across the classroom and increasing the ways in which knowledge is experienced and shared. Specifically, anti-oppressive practice counters power hoarding through leveraging all the expertise within the classroom, including and not limited to the professors, students, and teaching assistants (aqil 2021). Professors are also encouraged to invite guest lecturers who offer a wide variety of lived experiences that differ from academia to be a part of the teaching team, such as community members and organizations. These partnerships, when built intentionally, require appropriate compensation that reflects the time and effort provided to facilitate the course (Mitchell 2021). Last, but not least, is providing students with opportunities for experiential learning that allow them to be a part of the fabric of learning and hear from those who are experts in their lived experiences (Mitchell 2021). Through these varied approaches, power is diffused across the teaching teams, students, and communities, allowing learning to occur more organically and without a need for building an expertise on a topic.

Eliminating Paternalism

One example of paternalism in pedagogy is when instructors provide readings and source materials that only present a dominant worldview. Dismantling this form of paternalism involves faculty questioning their own assumptions about what constitutes representation and social justice by decentering sources that prioritize White-bodied, male, able-bodied, heteronormative scholarship (Manalo-Pedro et al. 2023). In our own experience, the interrogation by students of paternalistic syllabi can open up productive conversations about the historical and structural reasons for the exclusion of minoritized groups from academic scholarship. Thus, it is critically important to be deliberate about citing scholars of the global majority in course syllabi and in our work (Chakravartty 2018).

Questioning Objectivity

Questioning objectivity, or engraving subjectivity as a pedagogy practice, is an invitation to name and acknowledge that, as an instructor, you are not neutral in your thoughts or values. These things are present in your teaching style as well as the instructional design of your courses because of the meaning your worldview takes on in the classroom (hooks 1994).

Further, questioning objectivity invites instructors to take another look at how they plan to spend class time developing the practice of metacognition—that is, student reflection on how their worldview shapes their understanding of terms, processes, outcomes, and so on (Irvine 2020). Supporting students' individual and collective meaning-making also provides the opportunity for new definition development. As a pedagogy practice, this looks like a commitment to dialectic learning, critical reflection, and praxis (Irvine 2017). Curricularly, this could look like creating a team project, practicum, or capstone that allows students to apply what they learn in a real-world context, reflect on their learning as they go, and interrogate their previously held differences and how they evolved through field and group work.

Conclusion

bell hooks reminds us that the classroom is the most radical space of possibility in the academy, that education is a practice of freedom, and that teachers who believe in inclusive futures have the opportunity to reorient students toward more active and engaged participation in critical and transformative learning (hooks 1994). In this chapter, we argue that public health educators have a responsibility and must be well prepared to teach their students to work against systems of oppression that are present in public health. We agree with bell hooks that the classroom is an ideal space to model this work and demonstrate how power hoarding, paternalism, the commitment to the myth of objectivity, and a worship of the written word create inequities in the classroom that are perpetuated in "the real world," and further, can lead to poor health. We encourage public health educators to carefully consider and incorporate the anti-oppressive pedagogical and curricular shifts offered here so that their students have the preparation needed to interrogate, challenge, and change systems of oppression that negatively impact health and well-being.

References

Allen, Quaylan. 2015. "Race, culture and agency: Examining the ideologies and practices of US teachers of Black male students." *Teaching and Teacher Education* 47: 71–81.

Alsop, Elizabeth. 2018. "Who's teaching the teachers." *The Chronicle of Higher Education* 64: 23.

aqil, anushka. 2021. "Incorporating Anti-Oppressive Principles into Public Health Pedagogy: A Qualitative Inquiry." PhD diss., Johns Hopkins University.

aqil, anushka r., Mannat Malik, Keilah A. Jacques, Krystal Lee, Lauren J. Parker, Caitlin E. Kennedy, Graham Mooney, and Danielle German. 2021. "Engaging in Anti-Oppressive Public Health Teaching: Challenges and Recommendations." *Pedagogy in Health Promotion* 7 (4): 344–353.

Bentley, Kelly M., Deborah Fortune, Ronica Rooks, and Gayle Walter. 2021. "Antiracism and the Pursuit of Social Justice." *Pedagogy in Health Promotion* 7 (4): 296–298.

Brownell, S. E., & Tanner, K. D. 2012. "Barriers to faculty pedagogical change: Lack of training, time, incentives, and... tensions with professional identity?." *CBE—Life Sciences Education* 11 (4), 339–346.

Callaghan-Koru, Jennifer A., and anushka r. aqil. 2022. "Theory-Informed Course Design: Applications of Bloom's Taxonomy in Undergraduate Public Health Courses." *Pedagogy in Health Promotion* 8 (1): 75–83.

Campbell, Carolyn. 2003. "Anti-Oppressive Theory and Practice as the Organizing Theme for Social Work Education: The Case in Favour." *Canadian Social Work Review / Revue Canadienne de Service Social* 20 (1): 121–125.

Chakravartty, Paula, Rachel Kuo, Victoria Grubbs, and Charlton McIlwain. 2018. "# communicationsowhite." *Journal of Communication* 68 (2): 254–266.

Chandler, Caroline E., Caitlin R. Williams, Mallory W. Turner, and Meghan E. Shanahan. 2022. "Training public health students in racial justice and health equity: a systematic review." *Public Health Reports* 137 (2): 375–385.

Chávez, Vivian, Ruby-Asuncion N. Turalba, and Savita Malik. 2006. "Teaching public health through a pedagogy of collegiality." *American journal of public health* 96 (7): 1175-1180.

Clifford, Derek. 1995. "Methods in Oral History and Social Work." *Oral History* 23 (2): 65–70.

Collins, Patricia Hill. 2000. *Black Feminist Thought: Knowledge, Consciousness, and the Politics of Empowerment.* New York: Routledge.

Crenshaw, K. W. 1989. "Demarginalizing the Intersection of Race and Sex: A Black Feminist Critique of Antidiscrimination Doctrine, Feminist Theory and Antiracist Politics." *The University of Chicago Legal Forum* 1989 (1), Article 8, 139–167.

American Association of College of Nurses. n.d. "Curriculum Standards." About AACN. Accessed April 6, 2024. https://www.aacnnursing.org/about-aacn.

Dalrymple, Jane, and Beverley Burke. 2006. *Anti-Oppressive Practice: Social Care and the Law.* McGraw-Hill Education (UK).

Freire, Paulo. 2000. *Pedagogy of the Oppressed.* Continuum.

Giroux, Henry A., and David E. Purpel. 1983. *The Hidden Curriculum and Moral Education: Deception or Discovery?* McCutchan Publishing.

Grilo, Stephanie, Monét Bryant, Samantha Garbers, Maggie Wiggin, and Goleen Samari. 2023. "Effects of a Mentoring Program for Black, Indigenous, and People of Color and First-Generation Public Health Students." *Public Health Reports* 139 (3): 385–393.

hooks, bell. 1994. *Teaching to Transgress Education as the Practice of Freedom.* New York: Routledge.

Irvine, Jeff. 2017. "A Comparison of Revised Bloom and Marzano's New Taxonomy of Learning." *Research in Higher Education Journal* 33.

Irvine, Jeff. 2020. "Evaluating Fidelity of Implementation for a Powerful Learning Environment Classroom Intervention." *Journal of Instructional Pedagogies* 23.

Irwin, Ryan. 2022. "The Un-Essay, and Teaching in a Time of Monsters." *Teaching History: A Journal of Methods* 47 (1): 13–25

Jee-Lyn García, Jennifer, and Mienah Zulfacar Sharif. 2015. "Black Lives Matter: A Commentary on Racism and Public Health." *American Journal of Public Health* 105 (8): e27–e30.

Johnson, Azeezat, and Remi Joseph-Salisbury. 2018. "'Are you supposed to be in here?' Racial microaggressions and knowledge production in higher education."

Dismantling race in higher education: Racism, whiteness and decolonising the academy, 143–160.

Kalbarczyk, Anna, anushka r. aqil, Molly Sauer, Pranab Chatterjee, Keilah A. Jacques, Graham Mooney, Alain Labrique, and Krystal Lee. 2023. "Using Antioppressive Teaching Principles to Transform a Graduate Global Health Course at Johns Hopkins University." *BMJ Global Health* 8 (3): e011587.

Kim, Anatasia S., and Alicia Del Prado. 2019. *It's Time to Talk (and Listen): How to Have Constructive Conversations About Race, Class, Sexuality, Ability & Gender in a Polarized World*. New Harbinger Publications.

Kishimoto, Kyoko. 2018. "Anti-Racist Pedagogy: From Faculty's Self-Reflection to Organizing Within and Beyond the Classroom." *Race Ethnicity and Education* 21 (4): 540–554.

Koblinsky, Sally A., Katie M. Hrapczynski, and Jane E. Clark. 2015. "Preparing future faculty and professionals for public health careers." *American journal of public health* 105 (S1): S125-S131.

Kumashiro, Kevin K. 2000. "Toward a Theory of Anti-Oppressive Education." *Review of Educational Research* 70 (1): 25–53.

Lavallée, L. F. 2014. "Anti-oppression research." In *The SAGE encyclopedia of action research*, edited by Coghlan D., Brydon-Miller M., 41–44. Sage.

Leonardo, Zeus, and Ronald K. Porter. 2010. "Pedagogy of fear: Toward a Fanonian theory of 'safety' in race dialogue." *Race Ethnicity and Education* 13 (2): 139–157.

Lorde, A. 1984. *Sister Outsider: Essays and Speeches*. Crossing Press.

Lyons, Vivian H., Jessie Seiler, Ali Rowhani-Rahbar, and Avanti Adhia. 2023. "Lessons Learned from Integrating Anti-Oppression Pedagogy in a Graduate-Level Course in Epidemiology." *American Journal of Epidemiology* 192 (8): 1231–1237.

MacDonald, Judy E. 2008. "Anti-Oppressive Practices with Chronic Pain Sufferers." *Social Work in Health Care* 47 (2): 135–156.

Manalo-Pedro, Erin, Katrina M. Walsemann, and Gilbert C. Gee. 2023. "Whose Knowledge Heals? Transforming Teaching in the Struggle for Health Equity." *Health Education & Behavior* 50 (4): 482–492.

Mitchell, Tania D. 2021. "Critical Service Learning." In *Anti-Oppressive Education in Elite Schools: Promising Practices and Cautionary Tales from the Field*, edited by Katy Swalwell and Daniel Spikes, 85. Teachers College Press.

Mock, Brentin. 2020. "Dozens of City Governments Declare Racism a Public Health Crisis." *Bloomberg News*, July 13. https://www.bloomberg.com/news/articles/2020-07-13/dozens-of-cities-dub-racism-a-public-health-crisis.

Mohanty, C. T. 2014. "On Race and Voice: Challenges for Liberal Education in the 1990s." In *Between Borders: Pedagogy and the Politics of Cultural Studies*, edited by Henry A. Giroux and Peter McLaren, 145–166. London: Routledge.

Nescolarde-Selva, Josué Antonio, José-Luis Usó-Doménech, and Hugh Gash. 2017. "What Are Ideological Systems?" *Systems* 5 (1): 21.

Okun, Tema. 2021. "White Supremacy Culture: Still Here." May 2021. https:// socialwork.wayne.edu/events/4_-_okun_-_white_supremacy_culture_- _still_here.pdf.

Polston, Patsy M., Derrick D. Matthews, Shelley D. Golden, Carol E. Golin, Marissa G. Hall, Emmanuel Saint-Phard, and Alexandra F. Lightfoot. 2023. "Institutional Reform to Promote Antiracism: A Tool for Developing an Organizational Equity Action and Accountability Plan." *Preventing Chronic Disease* 20 (June): E50.

Sakamoto I, and Pitner R. O. 2005. "Use of Critical Consciousness in Anti-Oppressive Social Work Practice: Disentangling Power Dynamics at Personal and Structural Levels." *British Journal of Social Work* 35 (4): 435–452.

Strier, Roni, and Sharon Binyamin. 2013. "Introducing Anti-Oppressive Social Work Practices in Public Services: Rhetoric to Practice." *British Journal of Social Work* 44 (8): 2095–2112.

Witten, Nash A. K., and Gregory G. Maskarinec. 2015. "Privilege as a Social Determinant of Health in Medical Education: A Single Class Session Can Change Privilege Perspective." *Hawai'i Journal of Medicine & Public Health* 74 (9): 297.

Yee, J. Y., C. Hackbusch, and H. Wong. 2015. "An Anti-Oppression (AO) Framework for Child Welfare in Ontario, Canada: Possibilities for Systemic Change." *British Journal of Social Work* 45 (2): 474–492.

Chapter 10

Developing a Social Justice–Informed Curriculum for Public Health and Medicine

Tekisha Everette, Chelsey Carter, Amelea Lowery, and Danya Keene

Introduction

Social justice is at the core of public health's mission and values. It is well known that the health of the public is inseparable from the social conditions that foster health and illness, which are themselves produced by systems of unequal power. In the US, racism and other forms of structural discrimination are key drivers of population health, and efforts to achieve health equity will remain elusive without addressing these underlying forces of injustice (Yearby 2020). Racial injustice is a leading cause of premature death in the US, where Black-White mortality gaps are larger than the death toll caused by COVID-19 (Wrigley-Field 2020). At the same time, poverty, economic inequality, classism, and racial capitalism are major causes of premature morbidity and mortality (Bailey et al. 2017; Beech et al. 2021; Laster Pirtle 2020). Stigma and marginalization continue to undermine the health of LGBTQ+ individuals, despite recent reductions in structural forms of sexual-minority stigma (Hatzenbuehler 2014). Furthermore, individuals living at the intersections of multiple forms of oppression and stigmatization often experience unique health harms that are unaddressed by narrowly framed public health interventions (Bowleg 2012; Jackson and Mohr 2020).

Academic public health institutions that train future public health practitioners and researchers have a critical role and responsibility to play in addressing the public health crisis that racism and other forms of structural injustice produce (Takenaka et al. 2023). Yet, despite the deep historical connections between public health and social justice (Yong 2021), social justice public health pedagogy remains nascent. As of 2021, only six of fifty-nine

Tekisha Everette et al., *Developing a Social Justice–Informed Curriculum for Public Health and Medicine*. In: *Power, Privilege, and Public Health in the United States*. Edited by: Lorraine T. Dean and Keilah A. Jacques, Oxford University Press. © Oxford University Press (2025). DOI: 10.1093/9780197760956.003.0010 accredited schools of public health explicitly named social justice in their mission statements.

In 2016, the Council on Education for Public Health (CEPH) developed training requirements that address health equity and social justice by revising its foundational competencies. However, only one CEPH competency explicitly addresses racism and structural discrimination as a determinant of health, stating that students will "discuss the means by which structural bias, social inequities, and racism undermine health and create challenges to achieving health equity at organization, community, and society levels" (CEPH 2023). Other competencies mention health equity as a desired outcome of public health practice, without an explicit focus on systems of power and injustice that give rise to health inequities. For example, one competency requires that students "evaluate policies for their impact on public health and health equity," and another states that students will "advocate for political, social and economic policies that will improve health in diverse populations."

While CEPH's new competencies provide some impetus and direction for academic institutions to revise curricula to address racism and injustice, there is currently little pedagogical guidance on what it means to do this. For example, a recent systematic review found only eleven articles focused on training US public health students to address structural racism (Rosario et al. 2022). The literature also contains multiple and diverging definitions of what it means to take a social justice approach to public health (Gostin and Powers 2006). There is no unifying definition of social justice in public health, nor is there a unifying set of pedagogical goals or practices of educational competencies (Munala et al. 2023).

This chapter begins to explore this gap. We draw on the existing literature to develop a definition of social justice in public health and to identify characteristics of a social justice approach. We also draw on our own experience at the Yale School of Public Health (YSPH) to describe approaches to developing a social justice curriculum for Masters in Public Health (MPH) students across multiple fields and departments. While social justice curricula can often be siloed into certain courses or departments, we revised our core curriculum to ensure that all MPH students, regardless of their concentration, receive training in core social justice principles during their first semester at YSPH. Just as epidemiological and statistical training provide core tools that students carry forward and build on during their public health training, we argue that social justice frameworks should be a core foundation of public health pedagogy rather than an optional area of focus. Building on the foundation provided in this core course, we also developed a cross-departmental concentration and associated coursework that provides students with a deeper grounding and training in social justice approaches to advancing health equity in public health. Our new concentration is not alone. Between 2015 and 2023, several schools of public health developed cross-departmental concentrations with an explicit focus on social justice, with dozens more concentrations focused on health equity.

In the sections below, we first discuss different definitions of social justice in public health and develop our own definition that aligns with our curriculum at YSPH. We then discuss some key principles of a social justice approach that align with this definition. Finally, we discuss how we have applied our definition and characteristics to curriculum design at YSPH. Our intention is not to prescribe one definition or one approach but, rather, to provide an example of how explicitly defining social justice principles can guide public health pedagogy.

What Is the Definition of Social Justice in Public Health?

While thought to be core to the mission and values of public health, there is not a central definition of social justice in the public health discipline. Some existing definitions broadly define social justice, and others provide a narrowly tailored definition that is specific to public health. Prominent definitions of social justice in the public health discourse shape social justice either as an ethical consideration for the field—seemingly presenting it as tangential rather than core—or as an intractable component of and core approach to the work (Gostin and Powers 2006). Here are four varied definitions from a core textbook, the leading trade association for public health, a peer-reviewed article, and a theory-based book.

- Social justice is "the idea that all members of a society should be treated fairly and justly" (Birkhead et al. 2020).
- Social justice is "the view that everyone deserves equal rights and opportunities—this includes the right to good health" (American Public Health Association n.d.).
- "A public health perspective characterized by social justice argues that public health problems are primarily socially generated and can be predicted based on the level of injustice and inequality in a society. Thus, the solutions to such problems must be through progressive social and public health policies and are best understood as a collective responsibility shared across the various levels of society" (Wallack 2019).

- "A commitment to social justice, as we explicate it, attached a special moral urgency to remediating the conditions of those whose life prospects are poor across multiple dimensions of well-being. . . . A central social role of public health, grounded in social justice, is to draw attention to any aspect of the social structure that exerts a pervasive and profound effect on the development and preservation of health" (Powers and Faden 2006).

The variation found among these definitions is an indicator of the challenge the public health field has in incorporating and/or embedding social justice into the curriculum. Each of these definitions offers a different perspective on social justice and its meaning within public health and public health practice. Individually, the four definitions do not provide a complete narrative, and they each provide a different framing of social justice. As a collective, the definitions frame what social justice is and tell you how to achieve it. What is missing in this collective is naming what the root causes of injustice are and the imperative to act beyond analysis and education.

Our goal at the outset of our process to build a curriculum was not to create a singular definition of social justice. Definitions of social justice are multiple, and adding yet another did not seem to be of value. Rather, it was critical to frame a purposeful definition that centered on process, outcomes, and action; that could be tailored to multiple sectors of public health; and that could serve as the focal point of our curriculum. Thus, our definition of social justice in the public health context is that *everyone can attain good health and prevent illness and injury without socially created barriers. Achieving this requires recognition of the systemic and systematic challenges to health, a population and systems approach to addressing and redressing these challenges, and action to achieve and improve outcomes for individuals and communities. Socially just public health requires the foundational understanding that if any one person or community faces a greater burden than another based on societal/social actions and policies, we have failed in the mission of our field.*

This definition implores the field to analyze, understand, and act at systemic, population, and individual levels. It requires acknowledgement of historical and contemporary social ills that make good health unattainable, and it requires action toward correcting those ills as a core component of addressing the public's health. It mirrors the updated ten essential health services model by squarely positioning social justice back into the center of the field and not as a parallel factor of the work (Center for Disease Control and Prevention 2023). It defines success and failure and identifies the challenges that prevent success and promote failure. Ultimately, it is theoretical, aspirational, and actionable.

What Are Characteristics of a Social Justice Approach?

We used the above definition to guide the iterative development of our core MPH course entitled "Social Justice and Health Equity." This course was first launched in 2018 and was iteratively revised over the years in response to multiple forms of student feedback and refinement of social justice principles. The course is required of all MPH students at the Yale School of Public Health (YSPH). Most students take the course during their first semester at YSPH with the intention that they will apply social justice principles through the rest of their MPH studies and subsequent public health careers in diverse fields of public health research and practice, both in the US and in other global settings.

In recent years, we revised the course to center core principles of social justice that follow from the above definition. These principles are taught during the first class session and are then revisited and referred to iteratively throughout the semester. In launching a social justice program at their university, Munala et al. (2023) noted the need to explicitly identify and teach social justice principles, rather than assuming that all students have this background and a shared understanding. We had a similar experience. We also found that explicitly teaching core principles of social justice provided more opportunities for students to apply these core ideas to their unique areas of interest and the varying geographic contexts of their public health work. Below, we describe the core principles that we use to characterize a social justice approach: (1) upstream approaches, (2) attention to power, (3) attention to agency, resistance, and lived expertise, (4) reflexivity about our own role, and (5) movement toward equity.

Upstream Approaches

Taking a social justice approach requires us to look upstream to the root, or fundamental, causes of health inequity. If we only pay attention to concerns that are happening downstream, we will likely not get very far in addressing unequal burdens of health. Even worse, we may create or support a false narrative about the causes of inequities. Public health history is plagued by discourses of "personal responsibility" or "healthism" that blame individual behaviors or community dynamics for health inequalities that are rooted in structural conditions (Petteway 2021). Taking an upstream approach redirects attention to the manufactured structural conditions that produce health inequities.

More specifically, upstream thinking directs students' attention to forms of structural discrimination (e.g., racism, classism, sexism, and ableism) that are at the root of health inequities. Yearby (2020) presents a model that centers structural discrimination as an antecedent of social conditions (or social determinants of health), which are often the focus of health equity work. Yearby's model illustrates that attention to social determinants without attention to the structural discrimination that creates them, often through discriminatory laws and policies, falls short of conceptualizing the social production of health inequities. A social justice approach requires not just attention to the unequal social conditions that produce health inequities but attention to the forces that shape and recreate these unequal social conditions. In our required social justice and health equity course, we begin with Yearby's model to direct students' attention to root causes of inequality. We also introduce fundamental causes theory (Link and Phelan 1995) as a model to explain the ways that unequal structures of power, privilege, and resources shape and recreate health inequities across time, place, health outcomes, and disease risks.

Attention to Power

Power is at the heart of the *isms* presented in Yearby's model, at the root of fundamental cause theory, and at the top of the proverbial stream. We argue that taking a social justice approach requires attention to power structures and distributions of power that are at the root of health inequalities. In our core curriculum, we draw students' attention to power in multiple ways. First, we provide evidence of the ways that a lack of power creates unequal burdens of poor health outcomes. Drawing on fundamental cause theory, we illustrate how power shapes access to resources that are needed to avoid risk and the ways that racism and discrimination affect health through pathways of social and economic power (Link and Phelan 1995).

Second, we highlight the ways that systems of unequal power are self-serving. We acknowledge that race and racism are oppressive ideologies created to consolidate and maintain power. As Krieger (2020) articulates, race, sexism, heterosexism, and gender binarism are systems of "self-serving domination and privilege" that are created by people in power. Drawing on theories of racial capitalism, we discuss the ways that racism contributes to the accumulation of wealth and resources for White Americans. For example, we discuss the ways that racist housing policies and practices have created both burdens of housing insecurity for Black and Brown Americans and wealth for White Americans (Coates 2014; Taylor 2019). Similarly, we center power in our conversations around stigma, highlighting the ways that stigma works in the service of power to maintain existing inequities (Parker and Aggleton 2003).

We also discuss the ways that power is contested, drawing attention to the resistance, struggles, and triumphs of marginalized communities in the face of oppression and to the mutability of power dynamics across place and time. As policy scholars Michener and Ford (2023) note, researchers, policy makers, and advocates oriented toward advancing health equity should address racism and other structural determinants of health "with an eye toward the power resources and political assets of racially marginalized populations" (341).

Attention to Agency, Resistance, and Lived Expertise

Following from the factors described above, a social justice approach also requires attention to the agency, resistance, knowledge, and expertise of marginalized communities and commitment to practices that build on and uplift these community resources. Course material that introduces students to health disparities must clarify that these disparities exist despite powerful and skilled resistance. In our core MPH course, we include examples of activism, resistance, and collective action throughout our discussion of health inequities. We also introduce students to frameworks such as Sojourner Syndrome (Mullings 2005) and John Henryism that highlight the health costs of high-effort coping with and resistance to racism, gendered racism, and economic oppression.

Public health approaches that ignore agency, resistance, and lived expertise, can reinforce harmful stereotypes and unequal relationships of power. Additionally, public health approaches that ignore the long-time efforts of marginalized communities to "mitigate, resist, or undo" (Geronimus 2000) the harms caused by structural oppression may inadvertently undermine strategies that these communities have employed successfully to mitigate health inequities (Geronimus and Thompson 2004). Furthermore, public health efforts, including policy advocacy and reform, are likely to be more successful when they build on knowledge and expertise that exist within marginalized communities through participatory and collaborative approaches that recognize that those who are closest to the problem are closest to the solution.

As such, public health training must prepare future public health scholars and practitioners to prioritize and support community-based knowledge and expertise. In our core course, we introduce students to methods and principles of participatory research practices. We discuss techniques for and approaches to engaging stakeholders and building collaborative research agendas. We introduce students to methods that are grounded in community priorities, are rooted in local expertise, and are oriented toward using the knowledge gained through collaborative research to dismantle oppressive power structures (Daryani et al. 2022). We also take a critical lens, recognizing the ways that the growing prevalence of community-based participatory research (CBPR) at schools of public health can sometimes result in surface-level applications of these concepts that are not fully participatory and do not adequately address the challenges of working across power dynamics that often exist between public health institutions and those who experience the largest impacts of health inequities (Daryani et al. 2022).

Reflexivity about Our Own Role

A social justice approach to public health requires attention to the ways that public health researchers and practitioners (as individuals), public health institutions, and public health as a discipline all contribute to and are shaped by systems of structural inequality (Yearby 2020). As such, public health education programs must train students in the skills and habits of reflexivity. Reflexivity is a common practice among qualitative researchers who are trained to interrogate the way their own unique lenses shape their interpretation of data, and reflexivity is often a core component of qualitative method training. However, reflexivity should not be limited to qualitative research. Regardless of method, public health students should be taught to question and critically interrogate the ways that both their own individual lenses and broader systems of power shape their research questions, approaches, and analyses. Students should be taught to interrogate why certain methods are valued over others (Zuberi and Bonilla-Silva 2008); how society, economics, and power shape the burden of proof that is required of public health research; and why conventional wisdom is sometimes accepted without adequate empirical evidence when it serves the interests of those in power.

As others have noted, attention to reflexivity is a significant gap and limitation in public health education and is not addressed by CEPH competencies (aqil et al. 2021).

Reflexivity also requires attention to the history of public health, including how the discipline has participated in forms of racist, classist, sexist, and ableist policies and action. Students should be introduced to unethical and racist methods that have been used in public health practice (Hammonds and Reverby 2019) and to the ways that public health campaigns have participated in the production of racist and stigmatizing stereotypes (Burris 2002; Hardeman and Karbeah 2020). Students should also understand how public health data and knowledge can be appropriated and used to perpetuate oppression. For example, Swope (2023) describes how public health data and health equity goals were weaponized to support urban renewal and the appropriation of Black neighborhoods in Washington DC. Chapter 11 of this book is devoted to offering additional examples of how public health is used as a rationale for advancing oppression.

Movement Toward Equity

Finally, a social justice approach requires attention to praxis and to actions that move toward the shared goal of eliminating population-based health inequality. A starting point for this action is a shared understanding that any health difference between two socially constructed groups is unjust and must be reduced to zero. Movement toward equity must start with the explicit rejection of frames that overtly or subtly suggest that racial inequities, or inequalities created by other forms of oppression, are due to essential or innate differences or are acceptable at any levels. Along these lines, students should be trained to contextualize the health equity data they analyze for the root causes of structural discrimination to avoid inadvertently reinforcing harmful frames about the innate superiority of one group or another (Chowkwanyun and Reed 2020).

Moving toward health equity also requires a prioritization of equity as an outcome. Public health interventions and policies should be evaluated based on their ability to reduce disparities and to improve health for those who bear the largest burden of illness. Historically, as indicated by fundamental cause theory, new health advances tend to widen inequalities, as those with greater access to knowledge, resources, and power are better able to access and leverage these new advances (Glied and Lleras-Muney 2008). To avoid this outcome, interventions must intentionally and deliberately work to disrupt this exacerbation of health inequalities. As such, public health practitioners must be trained to identify barriers that disadvantaged groups may face in benefiting from new interventions or resources. Prioritization of equity also requires attention to unintended consequences of policies and programs that may seem to advance equity but, in reality, have the opposite effect.

Finally, moving toward equity requires that students are trained to translate knowledge into action. This requires teaching public health theories with a focus on praxis. In addition to providing students with standard public health training in intervention design, moving toward equity also requires preparing students with concrete skills in advocacy and activism that can be used to advance upstream changes to address structural drivers of health inequalities through policy change, organizing, and social movements. Public health training should also prepare students to engage in discursive or framing interventions that redefine health inequalities as problems of injustice and power inequalities.

Building a Social Justice and Health Equity Curriculum at the Yale School of Public Health: A Brief Case Study

In this final section we ask readers to consider, How do we train public health researchers and practitioners to take a social justice approach? What kind of pedagogical tools and courses are effective? And finally, what is the impact on student experience, student learning, student outcomes, student identities, and future careers? In the following section, we offer a brief case study that responds to these questions by following the core principles we described above: (1) upstream approaches; (2) attention to power, attention to agency; (3) resistance and lived expertise; (4) reflexivity about our own role; and (5) movement toward equity.

In 2018, a group of students and faculty at the Yale School of Public Health began a two-year collaborative planning process to develop a new cross-departmental concentration that focused on ameliorating health inequalities. This process was initiated by students who noted a lack of curriculum attention to health inequality within the US and a need for more integration of social justice frameworks into the MPH training program (despite the school's history of a strong focus on global health). The planning committee of students and faculty met to review existing programs at other institutions, discuss the broad goals of the concentration, develop the specific competencies it would address, identify existing elective courses, and create new coursework where significant curriculum gaps existed. Collaboration between faculty and students was central to the development of the concentration. Within the complex histories of institutional injustices, students emerge as integral leaders capable of catalyzing academia toward equity-focused pedagogy. This collaborative approach opens the door to uplift ideas that have not been tamped down by organizational barriers.

The new concentration, entitled the "US Health Justice Concentration" (Table 10.1) launched in the spring of 2021 with an inaugural cohort of seventeen students. In designing this new concentration, we focused on the characteristics of a social justice approach as outlined above. Students chose from a list of elective courses that provided upstream frameworks and attention to power structures (principles 1 and 2). We then developed specific coursework to address principles 3–5. As the Department of Social and Behavioral Sciences grew their faculty, specifically hiring faculty members with expertise in community-based research, health disparities, health equity, and structural racism, our course offerings blossomed to include additional courses dedicated to social justice and health equity. We offer a brief case study to describe these courses, their goals, and the programmatic and educational activities that derived from these courses.

Teaching Participatory Approaches

Our definition of a social justice approach highlights the importance of participatory research and action that acknowledge the expertise of historically marginalized communities and support initiatives that strengthen power and resources within these communities. As such, our concentration includes core coursework in community-based participatory methods. Community-based participatory research (CBPR) models have become the gold standard for engaging with socio-demographically diverse study populations and developing sustainable interventions that improve health outcomes in populations with health disparities (Goodman and Sanders Thompson 2017; Israel et al. 2005). To address this objective, Dr. Ijeoma Opara developed a course titled *Community-Based Participatory Research in Public Health*. This course provides an overview of the major theories, key principles, and strategies that CPBR can offer student researchers interested in effectively addressing health disparities from a bottom-up approach. Dr. Opara trains students on how to build meaningful relationships and partnerships with community members. Opara defines community members as individuals "who share a social, neighborhood, or cultural identity, and common resources (including geographic proximity), or communication channels (such as media, internet)" related to health and health outcomes. This course is not only salient to the MPH curriculum but attracts students from across university departments. Students in the course shared these reflections:

"This course should be essential for public health students. This course took the foundations of what we've learned in public health equity, social justice, and ethical practice and transformed them into actionable research skills. This is the kind of research practice that the new generation of public health researchers and professionals should not only be aware of but be skilled in enough to identify when there is inequitable overreach occurring in the researcher-participant relationship." (Student, Semester: Spring 2023)

"This class really taught me how to apply abstract concepts like intersectionality, reflexivity, and ethics. I learned how maintaining the rigor of research is not at odds with (and should answer to) uplifting the dignity of people and communities." (Student, Semester: spring 2022)

Participatory Approaches in Action

It was important that the concentration model the approaches that we are teaching our students. Like many well resourced universities and the economically distressed cities they inhabit, Yale University and the city of New Haven, Connecticut, have had a complicated relationship. The concentration has met these challenges head on, acknowledging the decades of divestment, capitalization on Black and Brown labor, and unethical health disparities that exist between those who are affiliated and protected by the university versus the New Haven community. One objective of the concentration is to redefine how students interact with the New Haven community and move away from models where students interact with community partners for short periods, often creating burden and not real impact. We envision building sustained relationships with community organizations that can create synergistic impact for our students and community partners. While we understand that transforming our school and the university's relationship with New Haven will not occur overnight, we are hopeful that these are the beginning steps toward repairing relationships between universities and their communities.

Disciplinary Critique and Reflexivity

A social justice approach to public health also requires and necessitates a critical lens to public health methodology, discourse, and practice. Inspired by the public health critical race praxis developed by Ford and Airhihenbuwa (2010), the concentration offers a seminar-style class for students to explore the intersections of knowledge, method, power, and justice through the lens of a specific public health topic. The course *Biomedical Justice: Public Health Critiques and Praxis* (taught by Professor Chelsey Carter) emboldens students to critique public health evidence, question public health practices, and develop health justice approaches. Professor Carter utilizes biomedicine not to simply signal a combination of biology and medicine, but rather, she deploys it as a framework that explains and helps students understand the unique cultural and philosophical commitments of Western culture's development of "medicine" and "public health" through global power dynamics. This is one of the concentration's most disciplinarily diverse courses, because we want to equip students with a toolkit of transdisciplinary approaches and perspectives when studying, identifying, and addressing these concerns. Students engage in critical social theory, anthropology, Black feminist health science studies, history of medicine, sociology, law, and science and technology studies. A student reflected, sharing, "I learned how to critique public health and biomedicine with a social justice, radical, Black feminist lens. Nothing will change unless public health practitioners actively fight against and critique the system from the inside" (Student, Semester: Spring 2023). All students are asked to consider their own positionality and think reflexively about how their own lived experiences shape how they will approach some of society's most vexing health concerns. Our curriculum, and especially this course, supports an environment where students can safely question, critique, and say the "wrong" thing as we work toward dismantling harmful beliefs about underrepresented communities. As one student remarked,

"I developed the ability to explain the influence of slavery and White Supremacy in how public health practice is today. I gained insight into how race is often used as a proxy for biology or behaviors and how this shapes the public health solutions we imagine. I gained insight into how the afterlife of slavery has impacted medicine, and how medicine impacts public health. I developed my knowledge about inequitable health in marginalized communities and how previous solutions have failed. I gained knowledge about authoritative knowledge and how that impacts public health approaches to solutions to health equity." (Student, Semester: Spring 2023)

Building Skills for Advocacy as a Tool for Equity

In keeping with the principle of moving toward equity, we designed a course titled *Advocacy and Activism* (taught by Professor Tekisha Everette) that provides students with frameworks and tools to be agents of change. The course centers on the important role of advocacy in public health and how public health practitioners, teachers, and students should use their expertise and learning to advocate for changes to the systems, policies, and practices that structure health inequalities. The course not only teaches students the theoretical approaches to community organizing, advocacy, and policy work but also helps students see how they can subvert traditional systems of knowledge through hands-on activism. One student shared that before taking this course, "I had no prior knowledge or experience in advocacy or activism. I think this class was one that I learned the most in due to the fact that I had no knowledge going into it. But also it broadened my understanding of advocacy and activism and made me realize that as public health professionals, no matter what the role, we all have a duty to advocate and/or participate in activism for the health of those in the US" (Student, Semester: Spring 2023). We've learned through this core course that many students long to put their public health skills into practice beyond the traditional research space. Giving students the opportunity to employ the skills of collective action and political activism through historical and intersectional lenses helps future public health practitioners understand why communities have been historically marginalized and underinvested. Assignments ranged from developing advocacy campaigns, conducting mock hearings, learning how to create a written testimony and how to present an oral testimony, and employing the intricacies of the legislative process at the federal, state, and local levels. A student remarked on the value of these skills, noting that it was

"…an essential course for anyone who plans to go into government work, policy, advocacy, lobbying, nonprofit work, anything connected in any way to policy and the US government. The primary project of developing an advocacy campaign was really fun and so educational. The Community Toolbox and other readings gave us structure for how to design an advocacy campaign, and class lectures and discussions clarified the process, so my group and I felt well supported and well prepared for writing our campaign plan. While before taking this course designing a campaign and engaging with the legislative process felt very overwhelming, now after taking this course I feel actually really confident in my ability to contribute to a campaign, figure out different stakeholders, learn about local political processes, and give written and oral testimony." (Student, Semester: Spring 2021)

Activist in Residence Program

Building on the Advocacy and Activism course, the department's new *Activist in Residence* pilot program (created and led by Professor Ijeoma Opara) brings to Yale activists from around the country who are engaging in current and impactful social justice issues that intersect with public health. The program seeks to advance the activist's platform, allow the activist to utilize the infrastructure and resources at Yale, and provide Yale students, faculty, and staff with the opportunity to work on social justice issues that impact public health. In the first year of the program, Professor Opara invited activist Angelo Pinto. Pinto is not only a veteran activist but also a lawyer, political strategist, and cofounder of Until Freedom, a nonprofit social justice think tank committed to police accountability and criminal justice reform. In 2022, students had the opportunity to learn from Professor Pinto and special guest lecturers at the intersection of incarceration, criminal justice reform, and community health. Guest speakers and panelists included Dr. Jamila T. Davis; Jackson, Mississippi, advocates Rukia Lumumba (People's Activist Institute, Electoral Justice League), Shawnee Benton Gibson, and Omari Maynard (Aftershock Documentary); and attorney Ben Crump. During the ongoing water crises

Table 10.1 Yale School of Public Health social justice curriculum

Course title	Units	Term
Required social justice coursework for all MPH students		
Social Justice and Health Equity	1	Fall
Required coursework for students in the US health justice concentration		
Advocacy and Activism	1	Spring
One of the following:		
Biomedical Justice: Public Health Critiques and Praxis	1	Spring
Community Based Participatory Research	1	Spring
One of the following practicum experiences:		
US Health Justice Practicum	1	Fall/spring
Summer internship (addressing relevant competencies)	0	Summer
Advanced Health Policy Practicum	1	Fall
Practice-Based Community Health	1	Spring
Health Policy and Health Care Management Practicum	1	Fall

One elective course that critically analyzes the roles of history, power, and privilege in creating and maintaining health inequities

One elective course that discusses how systems of government and law affect health equity at the local, state, and national levels

occurring throughout many poor and Black US cities, students were selected to participate in a community participatory action trip to learn about Jackson's public health crisis. This in-depth visit and engagement with residents helped students learn about the complexity of the public health crisis beyond water. Opportunities through the *Activist in Residence* program help students grapple with structural violence and create solution systems and focused solutions that get to the root of the problem and critically engage those most impacted. In the program's second pilot year, Activist-in-Residence Nelba Marquez-Greene (Walsh 2022) will center gun violence at the intersection of public health, focusing on mental health and trauma.

Conclusion

In the discussion above, we outlined some core principles, practices, and experiences associated with developing social justice pedagogy and curricula. We shared these as examples of how an explicit definition of social justice can be used to guide public health pedagogy with the ultimate goal of advancing health equity. Our definition and our approach are not intended to be prescriptive, as each program will need to develop curricula that align with its own student and faculty needs. At the same time, we hope to illustrate the importance of developing curricula around a shared definition of social justice with clearly articulated principles and reflections on the student impact of our courses.

We also acknowledge the limitations of the curriculum model we described above. Our model at YSPH provides all students with an introduction to social justice principles in a required core course and then provides an opportunity for students to dive deeper into these principles through a programmatic elective concentration. Preliminary qualitative feedback from students (collected through a variety of informal methods) identifies the gaps in this approach. Students expressed concerns that social justice principles were not integrated throughout the curriculum at YSPH. They argued that if social justice is at the core of improving the health of the public and if reducing health inequities is a priority of the discipline, then all subject matter should be taught through this lens.

We also must acknowledge that we provide a framework that is ultimately untested in its ability to advance justice and health equity. Just as public health interventions must be evaluated with respect to their impacts on equity, so too must curricula. As public health programs around the country develop curricula and programs centered on social justice, they must also develop plans to evaluate these programs with a focus on equity. We cannot assume the impacts of well-intended social justice pedagogy, especially given research showing that exposure to information about health disparities without appropriate framing can deepen stigma and stereotypes (Chowkwanyun and Reed 2020). Schools of public health must critically evaluate how social justice curricula shape student professional identity formation and future public health research and practice. Even the process of defining desired student outcomes will require conversation and thought.

Finally, we provided an example of curriculum development at one institution. Systemic change to incorporate social justice principles into public health education will require work across institutions, including possible revisions to CEPH competencies.

References

American Public Health Association. n.d. "Social Justice and Health." Accessed March 9, 2024. https://apha.org/what-is-public-health/generation-public-health/our-work/social-justice.

Aqil, Anushka R., Mannat Malik, Keilah A. Jacques, Krystal Lee, Lauren J. Parker, Caitlin E. Kennedy, Graham Mooney, and Danielle German. 2021. "Engaging in Anti-Oppressive Public Health Teaching: Challenges and Recommendations." *Pedagogy in Health Promotion* 7 (4): 344–353.

Bailey, Zinzi D., Nancy Krieger, Madina Agénor, Jasmine Graves, Natalia Linos, and Mary T. Bassett. 2017. "Structural Racism and Health Inequities in the USA: Evidence and Interventions." *The Lancet* 389 (10077): 1453–1463.

Beech, Bettina M., Chandra Ford, Roland J. Thorpe Jr, Marino A. Bruce, and Keith C. Norris. 2021. "Poverty, Racism, and the Public Health Crisis in America." *Frontiers in Public Health* 9: 699049.

Birkhead, Guthrie S., Cynthia B. Morrow, and Sylvia Pirani. 2020. *Turnock's Public Health: What It Is and How It Works.* Jones & Bartlett Learning.

Bowleg, Lisa. 2012. "The Problem with the Phrase *Women and Minorities*: Intersectionality—an Important Theoretical Framework for Public Health." *American Journal of Public Health* 102 (7): 1267–1273.

Burris, Scott. 2002. "Disease Stigma in U.S. Public Health Law." *Journal of Law, Medicine & Ethics* 30 (2): 179–190.

Center for Disease Control and Prevention. 2023. "10 Essential Public Health Services." https://www.cdc.gov/public-health-gateway/php/about/?CDC_AAref_Val=https://www.cdc.gov/publichealthgateway/publichealthservices/essentialhealthservices.html.

CEPH. 2023. "Council on Education for Public Health." 2023. https://media.ceph.org/documents/D2_guidance.pdf

Chowkwanyun, Merlin, and Adolph L. Reed Jr. 2020. "Racial Health Disparities and Covid-19: Caution and Context." *New England Journal of Medicine* 383 (3): 201–203.

Coates, Ta-Nahisi. 2014. "The Case for Reparations." *The Atlantic*, June 15, 2014.

Daryani, Poonam, Leila Ensha, Mariah Frank, Lily Kofke, Francesca Maviglia, and Alice M. Miller. 2022. "When Principles and Pedagogy Clash: Moving beyond the Limits of Scholarly Practices in an Academic-Community Partnership with Sex Worker Activists." *Global Public Health* 17 (10): 2500–2511.

Davis, Dána-Ain. 2019. "Obstetric Racism: The Racial Politics of Pregnancy, Labor, and Birthing." *Medical Anthropology* 38 (7): 560–573.

Ford, Chandra L., and Collins O. Airhihenbuwa. 2010. "Critical Race Theory, Race Equity, and Public Health: Toward Antiracism Praxis." *American Journal of Public Health* 100 Suppl 1 (Suppl 1): S30–S35.

Geronimus, A. T. 2000. "To Mitigate, Resist, or Undo: Addressing Structural Influences on the Health of Urban Populations." *American Journal of Public Health* 90 (6): 867–872.

Geronimus, A. T., and J. P. Thompson. 2004. "To Denigrate, Ignore, or Disrupt: Racial Inequality in Health and the Impact of a Policy-Induced Breakdown of African American Communities." *Du Bois Review: Social Science Research on Race* 1 (2): 247–279.

Glied, Sherry, and Adriana Lleras-Muney. 2008. "Technological Innovation and Inequality in Health." *Demography* 45 (3): 741–761.

Goodman, Melody S., and Vetta L. Sanders Thompson. 2017. "The Science of Stakeholder Engagement in Research: Classification, Implementation, and Evaluation." *Translational behavioral medicine* 7 (3): 186–491.

Gostin, Lawrence O., and Madison Powers. 2006. "What Does Social Justice Require for the Public's Health? Public Health Ethics and Policy Imperatives." *Health Affairs* 25 (4): 1053–1060.

Hammonds, Evelynn M., and Susan M. Reverby. 2019. "Toward a Historically Informed Analysis of Racial Health Disparities Since 1619." *American Journal of Public Health* 109 (10): 1348–1349.

Hardeman, Rachel R., and J'mag Karbeah. 2020. "Examining Racism in Health Services Research: A Disciplinary Self-Critique." *Health Services Research* 55 (Suppl 2): 777–780.

Hatzenbuehler, Mark L. 2014. "Structural Stigma and the Health of Lesbian, Gay, and Bisexual Populations." *Current Directions in Psychological Science* 23 (2): 127–132.

Jackson, Skyler D., and Jonathan J. Mohr. 2020. "Intersectional Experiences, Stigma-Related Stress, and Psychological Health among Black LGBQ Individuals." *Journal of Consulting and Clinical Psychology* 88 (5): 416.

James, S. A., D. S. Strogatz, S. B. Wing, and D. L. Ramsey. 1987. "Socioeconomic Status, John Henryism, and Hypertension in Blacks and Whites." *American Journal of Epidemiology* 126 (4): 664–673.

Krieger, Nancy. 2020. "Measures of Racism, Sexism, Heterosexism, and Gender Binarism for Health Equity Research: From Structural Injustice to Embodied Harm: An Ecosocial Analysis." *Annual Review of Public Health* 41: 37–62.

Laster Pirtle, W. N. 2020. "Racial Capitalism: A Fundamental Cause of Novel Coronavirus (COVID-19) Pandemic Inequities in the United States." *Health Education & Behavior* 47 (4): 504–508.

Link, B. G., and J. Phelan. 1995. "Social Conditions as Fundamental Causes of Disease." *Journal of Health and Social Behavior* Special Issue: 80–94.

Michener, Jamila, and Tiffany N. Ford. 2023. "Racism and Health: Three Core Principles." *Milbank Quarterly* 101 (S1): 333–355.

Mullings, Leith. 2005. "Resistance and Resilience: The Sojourner Syndrome and the Social Context of Reproduction in Central Harlem." *Transforming Anthropology* 13 (2): 79–91.

Munala, Leso, Elizabeth M. Allen, Oona M. Beall, and Kieu My Phi. 2023. "Social Justice and Public Health: A Framework for Curriculum Reform." *Pedagogy in Health Promotion* 9 (4): 288–296.

Parker, Richard, and Peter Aggleton. 2003. "HIV and AIDS-Related Stigma and Discrimination: A Conceptual Framework and Implications for Action." *Social Science & Medicine* 57 (1): 13–24.

Petteway, Ryan J. 2021. "Poetry as Praxis + 'Illumination': Toward an Epistemically Just Health Promotion for Resistance, Healing, and (Re)Imagination." *Health Promotion Practice* 22 (1_suppl): 20S–26S.

Powers, Madison, and Ruth R. Faden. 2006. *Social Justice: The Moral Foundations of Public Health and Health Policy.* Oxford University Press.

Rosario, Carrie, Saif Al Amin, and Cedric Parker. 2022. "[Un]Forgetting History: Preparing Public Health Professionals to Address Structural Racism." *Journal of Public Health Management and Practice* 28 (Suppl 1): S74–S81.

Satcher, David. 2005. "Introduction to Methods in Community-Based Participatory Research for Health." In *Methods in Community-Based Participatory Research for Health,* edited by Israel, Barbara A., E. Eng, Amy J Schulz, and E. A Parker, 3–26, San Francisco, CA: Jossey-Bass.

Swope, Carolyn B. 2023. "The Spatial Configuration of Segregation, Elite Fears of Disease, and Housing Reform in Washington, D.C.'s Inhabited Alleys." *Social Science History* 48(2): 173–201.

Takenaka, Bryce Puesta, Ying-Chiang Jeffrey Lee, Kene Orakwue, Hannah Aaron, Kelly Reyna, and Natalia Putnam. 2023. "Re-Imagining Public Health Education: Students' Perspectives and Considerations." *Health Education & Behavior* 50 (4): 477–481.

Taylor, K. Y. 2019. *Race for Profit: How Banks and the Real Estate Industry Undermined Black Homeownership.* UNC Press.

Wallack, Lawrence. 2019. "Building a Social Justice Narrative for Public Health." *Health Education & Behavior* 46 (6): 901–904.

Walsh, Joan. 2022. "'I Walk Into a Room and I Make People Cry': 10 Years After Sandy Hook." *The Nation,* December 13. https://www.thenation.com/article/society/nelba-marquez-greene-sandy-hook/.

Wrigley-Field, Elizabeth. 2020. "US Racial Inequality May Be as Deadly as COVID-19." *Proceedings of the National Academy of Sciences of the United States of America* 117 (36): 21854–21856.

Yearby, Ruqaiijah. 2020. "Structural Racism and Health Disparities: Reconfiguring the Social Determinants of Health Framework to Include the Root Cause." *Journal of Law, Medicine & Ethics* 48 (3): 518–526.

Yong, Ed. 2021. "How Public Health Took Part in Its Own Downfall." *The Atlantic,* October 23, 2021.

Zuberi, Tukufu, and Eduardo Bonilla-Silva. 2008. *White Logic, White Methods: Racism and Methodology.* Rowman & Littlefield.

Chapter 11
Historical and Contemporary Examples of Power, Privilege, and Public Health for Classroom Teaching

Lorraine T. Dean

Introduction

Racist and classist structures have been the backbone of US society and insidiously seep into how we study and teach health and medicine, how resources are funneled to support public health work, who is seen as a credible purveyor of scientific knowledge and decision-making, and how we execute public health interventions. As highlighted by the examples in this chapter, in many cases, preserving the health of the dominant White and wealthy population is used as a rationale for oppressive behavior.

These are not just historical incidents that are foundational to contemporary societal structures but are, rather, ongoing practices and structures that advance the belief that the health of some should be prioritized over the health of others. For example, US legislators have labeled books and curriculum like ours, which are founded in critical race theory, as a threat to health: in 2021, the Tennessee State Legislature, among others in other states, passed bills HB0580 and SB0623 (Tennessee General Assembly n.d.) to withhold funding from school districts and public charter schools that teach about structural racism and privilege. A few months later, Senator Marsha Blackburn penned an article (Blackburn 2021) about how a seven-year-old child in Tennessee felt so ashamed of being White after learning about critical race theory at school that the child's mother sent her for therapy citing, "She is depressed. She doesn't want to go to school." Senator Blackburn pitted the health of White children against the accurate teaching of the US's oppressive history, rather than acknowledging that anger, depression, outrage, and shame are reasonable emotions we should *all* experience in recounting the US's history

Lorraine T. Dean, *Historical and Contemporary Examples of Power, Privilege, and Public Health for Classroom Teaching*. In: *Power, Privilege, and Public Health in the United States*. Edited by: Lorraine T. Dean and Keilah A. Jacques, Oxford University Press. © Oxford University Press (2025). DOI: 10.1093/9780197760956.003.0011 of oppression. Bills like this contribute to the erasure of how oppression presently affects the health and well-being of those who are oppressed, as evidenced in the ongoing health inequities we see for minoritized persons in the US.

In other cases, attempts to exert power have been made at the detriment to the health of oppressed peoples and—in some cases—fatally so. For example, "Kill the Indian, Save the Man" was a refrain used to justify federally-funded Native American boarding schools in the late 1800s, designed to force Christianity and White American ideals onto Native American children (Solomon et al. 2022; Smith 2004). This form of cultural genocide was seen as a more economically feasible alternative to physical removal or killing of Native American populations (The Boarding School Healing Project n.d.). Some boarding schools received compensation per student, which incentivized overcrowding (The TRUTH Project 2023). Resultantly, they were rife with health and human rights violations, such as forced separations of families and children, inadequate food and medical care, sexual and physical abuse, and child labor—conditions that contributed to high rates of infectious disease and to the deaths of thousands of Native American children. Even as late as 2004, one child was found dead in a holding cell at Chemawa Boarding School in Oregon. The long-term impacts of these schools resound today as a historical trauma response that manifests in persistent mental, physical, and behavioral health disparities in Native American communities (Solomon et al. 2022).

We must reject the notion that scientific progress can occur without attention to equity and only accept progress when the benefits of health and medical science are equitably applied. It is not acceptable, nor is it a requisite proposition, that the health and well-being of some people are sacrificed to preserve the health and well-being of others. Chapter 3 of this book, on the coin of privilege, helps disrupt the frame of thought of trading privileges and thus will not be reprised here. Instead, this chapter will offer historical and contemporary examples of the ways in which preserving health has been used as a rationale for maintaining systems of privilege and oppression. Beyond these, there are many other examples across axes and dimensions of privilege. The scientific process (Zuberi and Bonilla-Silva 2008), scientific experiments, and public health policies are replete with examples of discrimination done in the name of scientific progress or public health advancement.

The remaining portion of this chapter cites examples, categorized under three domains, which can be highlighted as examples or case studies to be used in the classroom. The first section focuses on *public health education and medical training*, representing the ways in which public health training and practice institutions have been used to justify discrimination, oppression, and social exclusion. The second section focuses on *public health research* and how the advancement of public health knowledge has been considered a public health achievement even when it occurs at the expense of the health of oppressed peoples. The third section is about *public health policy* and offers examples of how both health and nonhealth policies have been used to justify preserving the health of some while denying the right to health for others.

While some examples are summarized here, the full stories behind them are embedded in historical and contemporary contexts, and they cannot be fully understood without acknowledging the context and societal norms of the time. In order to fully understand them, consider the lens of what was happening at that time and the US's social dynamics around issues of race, sexuality, labor, and gender at that time. These examples are not intended to be read with academic distance or with pity for those who experience oppression or marginalization. I am not a historian, and these examples are not new; however, these examples were selectively chosen to show how people use health and medical institutions and policies to exert power and privilege over others to produce discrimination, racism, social exclusion, and other forms of oppression. In using these as classroom examples, consider both health inequities caused by institutions or policies and effective ways to prevent or reduce their impact. Go beyond considering individual actions to consider what needs to happen at institutional or system levels to match the level at which these challenges are created.

For each set of examples, the reader is encouraged to reflect on the following:

- What health objective is being advanced?
- What are the characteristics of those whose health is being prioritized? In what ways do those compare or contrast with those whose health is being denied or overlooked?
- What oppressive persons (name them or their roles), systems, or historical precedents have allowed these events to happen?
- What could have been done differently to prioritize health equity?
- In what ways, if any, do we continue to contribute to the persistence of these oppressive systems? Who would need to act to change these systems, and what type of power do they need to have to effect change?
- What policies, programs, or social or material resources would be needed to redress or rectify these harms?
- What can you personally do or think about differently to avoid the persistence of or reproduce these forms of oppression?

Public Health Education and Medical Training

Power and privilege come into play for public health training in terms of (1) who gets trained, (2) what topics are taught and the lens through which they are taught, and (3) how training institutions are financed and accredited. Access to training at health and medical schools has traditionally been patterned by resources and privilege. Even the process of applying to health and medical higher education programs entails resources such as test preparation for required standardized tests (e.g., GRE and MCAT), application fees, and potentially taking on debt for tuition or for living expenses. Public health doctoral programs tend to admit students from high-ranking undergraduate schools that may have already had low numbers of underrepresented racial/ethnic minorities (URMs) and first-generation college students (National Academy of Sciences et al. 2011). In some cases, especially when there are family legacy preference programs, attending an elite institution may have been the result of privilege, not necessarily one's own talent or hard work. Then, when elite institutions favor those from other elite institutions, the cycle of inequality continues, which can exclude URMs and women, especially given that only 80% of URM doctorates receive degrees from high-prestige universities, versus 90% from well-represented groups and that women are more likely to land a faculty role at less prestigious institutions than where they were trained (Clauset et al. 2015).

These practices ultimately lead to the exclusion of voices in the academy—those people of color, women, and first-generation college students who have been systematically barred or discouraged from higher education—and create privilege gradients in purveyors of scientific knowledge. Even in this chapter, we acknowledge that the set of examples provided reflect gaps in scholarship on the health of Native Americans, Pacific Islanders, and Asian subpopulations—especially Southeast Asians—which experience health inequities. These voices may be excluded even when the research topic is focused on their experiences. For example, in 1936, the Carnegie Foundation wanted to advance research on "the infant race" but did not invite any Black scholars, citing that Black scholars would be too subjective and biased to study other Black people, an argument that White scholars studying White people were spared. Despite the availability of some of the most notable Black thinkers in US history, such as Zora Neale Hurston, W. E. B Du Bois, and Carter Woodson, the Carnegie Foundation instead hired a Swedish economist from outside the US, Gunnar Myrdal, who did finally include both White and Black scholars (Kendi 2016, 349). The practice of excluding voices from those who are from the communities being studied and who are experts in studying still persists (some would even say is rampant) in health and medicine research. Led by Dr. Elle Lett, a group of researchers has called out "health equity tourism," describing when "previously unengaged investigators [pivot] into health equity research without developing the necessary scientific expertise for high-quality work." Health equity tourism displaces resources that should go to scientists who are well informed and vested in the work, so as not to perpetuate unintentional harm (Lett et al. 2022).

Because bias is baked into our systems by virtue of excluding some voices while elevating others, we must be intentional to avoid reproducing these biases, which requires deliberate anti-oppressive action. The following example demonstrates how health and medical training that lacks an antiracist lens is actively harmful.

Example: Pathologizing Responses to Oppression

Chattel slavery of Black Americans in the US was the most heinous form and among the longest-lasting forms of slavery in the world, lasting hundreds of years (1619–1865) and leaving a legacy that is still felt today in US social norms, disparate health outcomes, and chronically higher and earlier mortality for Black Americans (Williams 2014). While the vast majority of African-descended people in the US were slaves up through 1865, there was a small percentage of "free Black" populations, which included people who had been freed or had purchased their own freedom from slavery. As of the 1840 census, the sixth decennial census in the US, 13.4% of Black people were free and 86.6% were enslaved (US Bureau of the Census 1975). This 1840 census was the first to attempt to capture the mental health status of respondents, enumerating the "number of insane and idiotic in public or private charge, by race."

Based on these census values, in 1842, Edward Jarvis, a Louisville-based psychiatrist published an article in the *New England Journal of Medicine*—among the most prominent medical journals at that time and still today, but one that also benefited from the chattel slave system (Jones et al. 2023)—citing that free northern-dwelling Black people were ten times more likely than enslaved southern Black people to be classified as "insane." He then erroneously concluded that "slavery has a wonderful influence upon the development of moral faculties and the intellectual powers; and refusing man many of the hopes and responsibilities which the free, self-thinking and self-acting enjoy and sustain, of course it saves him from some of the liabilities and dangers of active self-direction" and called for further research (Jarvis 1842). Just two months later, Jarvis published a retraction after realizing that the 1840 census numbers were incorrect (Jarvis 1842); however, by that time the rhetoric of slavery being good for mental health was already proliferating in the minds of purveyors of racism. He further attempted to press Congress to correct the census numbers, which never happened. Armed with the erroneous and racist interpretation of the erroneous data, two years later, the US secretary of state, John C. Calhoun, cited prevention of insanity as rationale for annexing Texas as a slave state (Jones et al. 2023; Rathbun 2001).

The belief that slavery and oppression were good for Black people was prevalent at the time, and in 1851, physician Samuel Cartwright introduced the phenomenon of "drapetomania" to describe a form of insanity that led Black slaves to run away from their heinous, enslaved conditions (Cartwright 1851). In each of these examples, responses to oppression were pathologized, as if the oppression itself was an inevitable part of life, and they omitted that freedom is fundamental to well-being. Pathologizing oppression further dehumanized Black persons, who were only having reasonable physical and emotional responses to oppression.

Echoes of these historical examples reverberate in contemporary society. Even in 2023, as we develop this book, this false rhetoric of the benefits of oppression to those who are oppressed continues to be espoused. In late July 2023, the Florida Board of Education approved a new social studies curriculum that claimed that enslaved Black Americans "developed skills which, in some instances, could be applied for their personal benefit." This same rhetoric is now being applied to other populations that have experienced oppression: in a debate about these standards on a conservative news outlet, a media personality paralleled how the skills that some Jewish people learned during the Holocaust may have preserved their lives, as they were useful to Nazi leaders (Vinokour 2023).

In earlier periods of the US Civil Rights Movement in the 1960s (we are still in a Civil Rights Movement in the US), schizophrenia was cited as the root of racial protests about Black inequality. In 2020, during the Black Lives Matter protests due to unjust police killings of Black people, some news outlets framed racial protests as "riots," which hinted at crazed behavior rather than a reasonable response to structural violence committed against people (Blain and Zoellner 2020). In contrast, throughout US history, many of the same riot behaviors have been used to advance labor movements and women's rights movements (Zinn 2005), yet when race-based protests occur, Black mental health is to blame.

Had these scientists used an antiracist lens, conclusions that blamed the victims' mental health for reasonable responses to oppression would have been considered nonsensical; Jarvis's conclusions would have raised immediate flags and might never have been published. A racist belief system also stymied the assessment of how various levels of oppression, such as White indentured servitude that ran alongside chattel slavery, might have contributed to poor health.

Example: Accreditation Weaponized: The Flexner Report and the Pruning of Historically Black Medical Schools

Throughout US medical history, White self-interest has been at the heart of driving how public health and medical training institutions have been set up. This is apparent in the story of the 1910 Flexner report that led to the closing of the majority of historically Black medical schools (Flexner 1910). At that time, germ theory was the predominant disease distribution theory and shaped the curriculum and approach to both medical and public health training at the time (Krieger 2000). Even germ theory was tinged with a racist lens: British surgeon Joseph Lister and bacteriologist Louis Pasteur in the 1860s recognized that "germs have no color line" and that the infections moving through Black populations, especially Black domestic help in White homes, could put White populations at risk (Gamble, 1995). It was these fears of contagion from Black to White communities that drove efforts to train Black physicians, albeit in a limited way that was focused on hygiene and disease containment rather than preserving the overall health of Black people. Due to Jim Crow laws enforcing segregation of health facilities (Plessy v. Ferguson 1896; Pollard 2012), the care for the nearly 10 million Black Americans would largely fall on Black physicians trained at Black medical schools (Miller and Weiss 2012), making Black medical schools a cornerstone for advancing Black health.

In 1909, the philanthropic Carnegie Foundation set a charge to improve the nation's health by focusing on improving the quality of medical education. At that time, medical education was based on a for-profit model that led to a large number of poorly trained physicians (Duffy 2011). Thus, the Carnegie Foundation hired Abraham Flexner, a White male educator (not a physician), to survey 155 medical schools in the US and Canada and to generate a report on the quality of those schools (Steinecke and Terrell 2010). Historians now recognize that the study may have also been covertly funded by the Association of American Medical Colleges (AAMC), which had a vested interest in protecting the finances of physicians by limiting the size of the physician workforce (Miller and Weiss 2012). The standards that Flexner set in his report were largely based on influences from German medical education (which were being promoted by his colleagues and advisors), which was focused on scientific research, with financing models based on philanthropically funded research rather than medical education, training, and patient care (Duffy 2011).

Flexner's report evaluated medical schools based on the rights and resources those schools had in relation to the embodying university, admission standards, physical facilities and having well-equipped laboratories, and instruction by physician scientists. He rated medical schools into three categories, based on a referent category of Johns Hopkins medical school, which he considered the gold standard; he himself had trained as an undergraduate at Johns Hopkins University, and many of his advisors at the time of his evaluations were Hopkins-affiliated, including the founding dean of Johns Hopkins. Under these standards, the seven Black medical schools had little recourse from harsh evaluations. Black medical schools did not have the resources (due to keeping tuition affordable for Black students) or endowments that predominantly White-serving medical schools had and were often funded through church donations or other charitable giving. Thus, when the Flexner Report was issued, five of the seven Black medical schools were considered substandard and were later recommended for closure.

The only two that survived were Howard and Meharry medical schools, which Flexner deemed as credible and sustainable (Laws 2021). In his two-page addendum that focused on Black medical schools, he suggested that Black students should be well trained but with more restricted emphasis on hygiene rather than therapeutic treatments, like surgery (Laws 2021). Even so, implementing the recommended training would be an outsized expense for already underresourced Black medical schools, given the Flexner report's overall recommendations that medical schools have large and expensive laboratory facilities and integrate hospital-based training into medical education (Laws 2021). In order to achieve the new standards set forth by the Flexner report, both Meharry and Howard requested resources from the Carnegie Foundation and were summarily denied. Further, the Flexner report offered no recommendations for targeted strategies or how other entities, such as the federal government or other organizations, could help rectify inequities in medical school training facilities. In fact, Flexner endorsed that given the social and economic position of Black Americans, "inequalities must be tolerated" and seemed resigned that Black physicians might not meet ideal standards and Black patients would be relegated to "the best type of physician so distributable." He explicitly framed the need for high-quality Black medical education in terms of White self-interest: "The negro must be educated not only for his sake, but for ours. He is, as far as the human eye can see, a permanent factor in the nation. He has his rights and due and value as an individual; but he has, besides, the tremendous importance that belongs to a potential source of infection and contagion" (Steinecke and Terrell 2010; Flexner 1910). While his personal beliefs and racist intentions are debated (Miller and Weiss 2012), the overall rhetoric at the time was still premised on racial inferiority of Black people, and his report was easily weaponized to promote the closure of the majority of the extant Black medical schools.

The impact of the Flexner report is still felt today, over 120 years later. Scholars like Dr. Vanessa Northington Gamble have documented how hospitals for Black people have evolved over history and how that history affects contemporary physician workforce trends and Black health disparities (Northington Gamble 1995). Recent studies have quantified how the closure of Black medical training facilities has affected the Black medical workforce. In 1970, the Association of American Medical Colleges (AAMC) set a goal of 12% for Black medical student enrollment, which still has not been met fifty years later (Campbell et al. 2020). The AAMC documented that a hundred years after the Flexner report (in 2010), the proportion of Black physicians to the Black US population was actually lower than it was in 1910, when the Flexner report was issued (Steinecke and Terrell 2010). By 2018, only 5% of the US Black population were trained physicians, representing a pitiful 4% increase over the past 120 years and largely driven by an increase in Black women physicians, with no statistically significant change in the percentage of Black male physicians (Ly 2022). A simulation estimated that 27,773 Black graduates could have entered the workforce between the time the schools closed and 2019. Had the five closed schools remained open, they estimate a 29% increase in the number of graduating Black physicians in 2019 alone (Campbell et al. 2020).

Despite the setbacks that the Flexner report had on Black medical training and access to healthcare for Black people, Black Americans showed their resilience. The timing of the closure of these medical schools was especially unfortunate given the flu epidemic that reached the US in 1918 killed an estimated 1 million people in the US. Black Americans actually had lower flu morbidity than the general population (due in part to greater exposure to earlier waves and a less virulent strain that conferred protective benefits and in part to racial segregation that may have unintentionally quarantined Black Americans) yet higher mortality, attributed in part to poor access to quality healthcare. In community-driven responses, Black nurses, Black churches, women's groups, newspapers, and community leaders promoted education and prevention and mobilized local volunteers to provide home-based care (Krishnan et al. 2020).

Later, Black community groups continued to stand in the gap for poor health care access for the Black community: for example, the Black Panthers' establishment of free community health clinics (Bassett 2016).

Public Health Research

Issues of power and privilege are through lines of public health research, from who produces knowledge and the lens they bring, to what types of questions are asked, to what's considered credible evidence and ethical research practice.

The privilege gradients in who are purveyors of scientific knowledge are well documented. A US national survey of 7,024 academic faculty in social and physical sciences and humanities from 2017 to 2020 found that faculty were up to 25 times more likely to have a parent with a PhD than the general population—and this rate nearly doubles at the most prestigious institutions and has been stable across the past 50 years (Morgan et al. 2022). It begs the question: How do academic researchers, who tend to be from the highest levels of privilege, learn to serve people who tend to be from the lowest levels of privilege?

We must also examine how privilege and positionality biases frame our scientific questions: you can't ask racist (or sexist or homophobic) questions and expect antiracist (or antisexist or antihomophobic) answers. For example, some of my previous work focused on exercise interventions for people with a history of cancer, and many people were interested in how well these exercise interventions worked for various subpopulations. Often, people would propose questions like "Are there racial differences in performance in exercise interventions for people with a history of cancer?" However, this question automatically sets up for conclusions that blame people's racialized status for their performance and can lead to conclusions such as "Asian people perform worse than White people on the intervention." It also leaves us with no actionable remedies, as we cannot modify how someone's racialized experience has played out in their lives (though we can attempt to address or remediate racist experiences). Instead, an antiracist reframing of this question would be "Does the exercise intervention have equal benefit to people of different racial groups?" This reframing refocuses the question on the actual challenge: that our interventions may be designed with our privilege and bias baked in and that, if there are differences, it is due to the defaults of the intervention, not due to the identity of the participant. The reframing also changes the target to examining the modifiable features of the intervention that might need to be changed to have equal benefit. Carla Goar's chapter in Tukufu Zuberi's book *White Logic, White Methods* lists several examples of how the experimental method has been used to justify discrimination, asking questions that are inherent with bias (Goar 2008).

The reframing also influences the populations that become the focus of research. For example, our explanations for racially motivated acts of violence are often attributed to unhinged individuals who espouse supremacist beliefs, without acknowledgment that those individuals are emboldened by communities of race supremacists who go unnamed. For that reason, we do not sufficiently name race supremacists as a population to study or intervene upon and have failed to define and differentiate racial supremacy groups who seek to oppress, like the Ku Klux Klan and American Identity Movement, from racial pride groups, like the Black Panthers, who sought to improve the health of both Black people and others (Bassett 2016; Morabia 2016).

Privilege even frames what is considered credible to be counted in the course of scientific study; consider what your reaction, as a reader, would have been had the previous paragraphs not included quantitative statistics to support their arguments. Things that are discrete and can be counted are prized—not that we should discount them, but this value reflects what we choose to count and how that reflects our privilege. For example, in studies of health and social capital, low voting registration rates have been used to represent low social capital in Black neighborhoods (Dean and Gilbert 2013; Gilbert et al. 2022); however, the decision to use voting registration as a measure of social capital itself reflects having the privilege of being part of a social group to whom voting is accessible. In the US, Black voters have been historically and contemporarily disenfranchised or altogether barred from participation, so using voting rates to measure social capital embeds this biased system. Instead, Black communities may have other unique forms of social capital, like faith groups, cookouts, or block parties (Dean et al. 2015), which may be better used to count social capital.

Privilege frames our research ethics and what is considered to be ethical research practice in terms of our target populations, our incentives for participation (or lack thereof), and our conclusions. As previously mentioned, we cannot have true scientific progress without attention to equity. The examples below recount how those who have racial privilege in the US have sacrificed the health of less privileged groups in the name of scientific advancement.

Example: Trading Humanity for Scientific Advancement

The US has a long history of unethical experimentation, with one of the most notable and egregious examples being the Tuskegee Syphilis Study (Gamble 1997; Thomas and Quinn 1991). Even after the legal end of chattel slavery by the Emancipation Proclamation in 1863 and the 13th Amendment to the Constitution in 1865, Black bodies continued to be used unethically for experimentation in US hospitals (LaVeist et al. 2000). Even in death, Black bodies were abused in the name of scientific advancement, through grave robbing of Black and Native American cadavers for medical experimentation (Dula 1994) or unauthorized use of their biological data, as in the case of the Henrietta Lacks cell line (Baptiste et al. 2022). Lesser known are some of the unethical experiments conducted on Black prison inmates, reflecting failures in both the health and carceral systems that were supposed to protect them.

As chronicled in the book *Acres of Skin* (Hornblum 2013), Holmesburg Prison near Philadelphia was the site of the atrocious unethical experimentation on three hundred mostly Black male inmates—and the race of the inmates likely contributed to the lack of protest that allowed these experiments to continue for nearly twenty-three years. Holmesburg Prison primarily housed incarcerated persons from the nearby inner city Philadelphia areas that were associated with high crime and recidivism rates; however, these areas were also those that were most devoid of investment of city resources, and the prison became a symbol of the city's approach to criminalizing poverty rather than putting resources toward eradicating it (MacLure 2021). Prison experimentation was common and considered ethical at the time, on the grounds that it allowed prisoners to make money and do a public service that would help repay their debt to society due to the harms their crimes had caused (MacLure 2021); nonetheless, the expected standards for ethical conduct were not followed in the Holmesburg cases.

In 1951, Dr. Albert Klingman, a faculty member at the University of Pennsylvania Department of Dermatology, was called to the prison to initially treat an outbreak of athlete's foot. Up through the 1970s, he engaged in a lucrative practice of experimentation on Holmesburg inmates who he described as "natural resources of scientific advancement." While done in the name of dermatological science, in actuality, they exploited resources for his personal gain and professional advancement: Dr. Klingman received academic rewards, including publications in prestigious journals such as *Archives of Dermatology, JAMA*, and the *Journal of Investigative Dermatology* (Bigby 1999) and financial incentives from thirty-three pharmaceutical companies and agencies, including Johnson & Johnson, Dow Chemicals, and the US Army (Brown and Sarisohn 2022).

During the Holmesburg Prison experiments, prisoners were subjected to testing of chemicals and medications from cosmetic and pharmaceutical companies, viruses, fungi, asbestos, and chemical agents. Inmates were exposed to herpes, poisonous skin-blistering chemicals, including dioxin—used in Agent Orange—and radioactive isotopes. Klingman went so far as to remove inmates' thumbnails to infect them with ringworm (Brown and Sarisohn 2022). While participants consented and were paid, the process of recruitment was coercive. Most of the inmates did not have literacy, and risks were not explained such that informed consent could be obtained. Most of the incarcerated were still awaiting trial, and the prison played on their poverty and desperation for bail money, paying them $1 per day to get them to agree to these abusive experiments (Brown and Sarisohn 2022).

Further, the research suffered from incomplete data collection, tested scientific questions of questionable beneficence, and exposed participants to unnecessary risks. The US Food and Drug Administration investigated the experiments in 1966, but experiments continued until 1974, when they were finally shut down by the Philadelphia prison's board of trustees after complaints, community protest, and personal testimony of abuse from inmates who had been in Klingman's experiments (MacLure 2021).

The victims of these experiments had long-term health risks and challenges, which they believe originated from these experiments. In 2000, a group of victims called "the Experimentation Survivors" used this as the foundation for a lawsuit against Klingman and the University of Pennsylvania to receive financial remuneration and access to medical care. Even then, they did not find justice or redress. Due to a two-year statute of limitations, which would have required them to file a lawsuit while they were still in prison, the lawsuit was thrown out (MacLure 2021; Brown and Sarisohn 2022). Instead, the mayor of Philadelphia issued a formal statement of apology in 2022, the University of Pennsylvania removed Klingman's name from honorific events, and the university set aside funds for fellows to study dermatological issues in Black and other people of color (Associated Press 2022). Many of these men are still alive and continue to live with long-term debilitating conditions, with no remuneration or redress.

Example: Research for "Progress," Not People: The Institutionalization of Racism in the Red Lake Nation Experiments

A group of Native American researchers recently published the "TRUTH Project Report," which chronicles the Red Lake Nation experiments by University of Minnesota (UMN) investigators, which occurred from 1953 to 1971. Building on a series of research studies of the Red Lake Nation children, initially in response to seasonal outbreaks of acute kidney infections among children believed to have been caused by streptococcal skin infection, in 1971, Dr. Lewis Wannamaker, faculty member at UMN, led a series of studies focused on the use of penicillin to treat strep-related impetigo skin conditions (Ferrieri et al. 1973). There was already a strong body of research suggesting that long-acting penicillin was effective at preventing strep infections in military personnel; however, researchers argued that there was limited evidence about penicillin's effectiveness "in populations at high risk, such as the one at Red Lake Nation." In the name of advancing science that could benefit military personnel, not just anyone with strep, these researchers used the children at Red Lake Nation as a testing lab (Ferrieri et al. 1973; The TRUTH Project 2023).

In several controlled and crossover design studies, seventy-eight children from eighteen families were enrolled and followed to assess how the use of penicillin, and particular doses of penicillin, might prevent new skin lesions within a six-week follow-up period (Ferrieri et al. 1973, 1974). After the publication of the studies, the UMN Committee Against Racism (CAR) issued reports documenting these experiments, titled "Exploitation on Red Lake Indian Reservation" and "Medical Research for the U.S. Military Carried out on the Red Lake Indian Reservation" (The TRUTH Project 2023) and called out the racist beliefs on which the experiments were founded. They were unwilling to entertain Dr. Wannamaker's rebuttals of the report, citing that "the intentions of the health CAR are to stop the racist research by working with the Indian Community, and to work with them to eliminate the impetigo problems from the children. This illustrates the institutionalization of the racism, because when a volunteer organization has to eliminate a problem that a professional team of investigators has been paid ½ million dollars to study, something is wrong, with the research itself, the granting institutions, or the health care institutions, etc" (The TRUTH Project 2023). The CAR appropriately called out yet another way in which research has been exploitative, by focusing on identifying and studying a health problem without a commitment to healing the problem in the community, sometimes leaving it to external organizations who are less resourced to actually resolve the problem.

Public Health Policy and Practice

Public health policies come in many forms and at various levels—ordinances, laws, mandates, and statutes at the local, state, and federal levels—and in some cases are used with explicit intent to discriminate. Sometimes they are explicit about protecting the majority population, as in former US President Donald J. Trump's 2016 presidential campaign comments about immigrants to the US from Mexico: "They're sending people that have lots of problems. . . . They're bringing drugs. They're bringing crime." In linking foreign-born persons to substance use and crime, he was invoking a health argument designed to protect a White majority. Later, he made a 2019 proclamation for consular officers deny visas to immigrants seeking to live in the US, unless they can prove that they "will be covered by approved health insurance" within thirty days of entering the US and that they have "the financial resources to pay for reasonably foreseeable medical costs." The former president used the rationale that legal immigrants are three times as likely as American citizens to be lacking health insurance and that "immigrants who enter this country should not further saddle our health care system, and subsequently American taxpayers, with higher costs" (Shear and Jordan 2019). This was reversed by President Joe Biden in 2021 and is no longer enforced (Chalfant 2021).

Discriminatory intent or impact may be coded as protection against health risks, often invoking limiting the spread of disease—for example, in the US in the early 1900s, when containing the spread of tuberculosis was used as a front for residential segregation. Over time, proponents of discrimination have become savvier and at times reframed discriminatory actions as a way to protect the health of oppressed populations, as in the case of the forced sterilization of Black women (Price et al. 2020) and incarcerated Black and Latina women (Nuriddin et al. 2020) and as in the example in the next section, of containing the spread of tuberculosis in Baltimore, Maryland.

Other times, public health policies can themselves limit access to health or promote health and health equity. For example, in 2018, Arkansas became the first US state to implement work requirements for healthcare access

through Medicaid. Within just six months of the enactment of this requirement, there was a 12% reduction (~17,000 people) in Medicaid coverage, a
significant increase in the percentage of uninsured persons, and no impact on
employment, even though 95% of the people affected by the policy already
met the requirement or were exempt from it (Sommers et al. 2019). In
contrast, the passage of our contemporary Medicare system by President
Lyndon B. Johnson in the 1960s largely led to the racial desegregation of
hospitals. As required by Title VI of the Civil Rights Act, passed in 1964,
federal funding was withheld from hospitals that racially segregated patients.
There was a swift and positive response; within just four months over 1,000
hospitals became desegregated (Sternberg 2015). This noteworthy example
shows how public health policies can help to dismantle structural racism and
discrimination—something we should strive to do with more public health
policies.

Policies about health may intersect with other systems, including the
carceral, education, and housing systems. For example, Dr. Julia Raifman
has several studies showing that laws that criminalize same-sex marriages are
adversely associated with sexual minority youth's mental health and higher
suicide rates. While these laws are not framed to be about health, their
discriminatory impact is detrimental to health.

In other cases, a failure to provide healthcare, and instead stigmatize or
criminalize those in need of healthcare, has been used to oppress people or
enforce privilege gradients. The examples below show the ways in which both
health and nonhealth policies have been used to discriminate and oppress.

Example: Weaponizing Public Health Policies to Discriminate and Oppress

In the early 1900s, tuberculosis (TB) was among the deadliest communicable
diseases in the US, killing 194 per every 100,000 persons, with race-based disparities in mortality outcomes (Doege 1965). In 1904, Baltimore, Maryland,
hosted the nation's first conference on TB, attracting thousands of people.
The Baltimore City Health Department showcased photographs and maps of
TB mortality, revealing that the predominantly Black area of Druid Hill Park
had troublingly high rates of TB—troubling because of the threats posed to
Baltimore's White population. This area, which housed working-class Black
people who were often domestic workers in White homes, who would be seen
as vectors of disease to White families, was labeled the "Lung Block" and had
a TB death rate seven times higher than the general city rate (Roberts 2003;

Nuriddin et al. 2020). With these maps, Baltimore's Lung Block became "a symbol for Black disease" (Roberts 2003), and TB containment became the way in which public health policies were weaponized to restrict the movement of Black bodies in the city.

In *The Black Butterfly*, Dr. Lawrence Brown details how sanitation laws in Baltimore were used as grounds for racial segregation (Brown 2021). In the early 1900s, prompted by fears of a "Negro invasion" after a Black Yale graduate and three additional Black families moved into a previously all-White neighborhood in Baltimore, Mayor John Barry Mahool signed the nation's first set of anti-Black racial zoning laws, at times claiming that they protected health: "Blacks should be quarantined in isolated slums in order to reduce the incidence of civil disturbance, to prevent the spread of communicable disease into nearby white neighborhoods, and to protect property values among the White majority" (Rothstein 2015, as cited in Loyola University Maryland 2019; Power 1983). In 1917, the US Supreme Court deemed Mayor Mahool's 1911 ordinance unconstitutional, not on the basis of Black discrimination, but because it restricted White homeowners' choice of to whom to sell (Loyola University Maryland 2019).

Baltimore's next mayor, James H. Preston, ran on the platform of continuing the crusade to maintain segregation in Baltimore, also invoking the health argument. To circumvent the Supreme Court's ruling on Mahool's racial zoning law, he implemented a rule requiring city building inspectors and health department investigators to issue code violations to homeowners who rented or sold to Black homebuyers in White neighborhoods (Loyola University Maryland 2019). In February 1917, Preston convened a group of Baltimore physicians, social workers, and concerned citizens to address the death rate of Black Baltimoreans due to TB. Cleverly, Preston now reframed the need for policies that displaced a segment of Black people to a colony outside Baltimore as important for the health of Black people, though all prior indications of intent suggested that the motivation for these segregation policies were to protect White Baltimoreans. It was a convenient argument that also served the purpose of appeasing White fears of the "Negro invasion." Preston's plans were thwarted due to the annexation of the area that would have become the Black colony. Even though both Preston and the Baltimore Health Department recognized that the unsanitary social conditions that Black people were exposed to and the derelict conditions of sewers and alleys allowed TB to proliferate, his administration continued to claim that exposure to Black people was the cause of the spread of TB and that race-based quarantine would be necessary for the protection of White health. The local newspaper, the *Baltimore Sun*, advanced these racist arguments by stating that Black people "constituted a menace to the health of the White population" (Staff Writer 1918). In addition to showing how local policies, in the name of preserving public health, can be weaponized, this also shows how media and other domains of society can also be weaponized.

Protection from infectious disease continues to be used to discriminate. For example, at the height of the COVID-19 pandemic, fear of the spread of infection in Native American communities led one New Mexico hospital to put into place an "undisclosed policy" that separated indigenous mothers from their newborns (Furlow 2020), an act of racial profiling.

Example: Criminalizing the Healthcare System's Inherent Failures

The US has a history of criminalizing its own practice of withholding healthcare. In the case of Black people with mental health conditions, the US has at times failed to hospitalize Black people and instead held them in prison, segregated them in underresourced mental facilities, or in the past fifty years, locked them away in correctional facilities or public psychiatric hospitals that have not had adequate treatment resources (Geller 2020).

One glaring example of how the lack of mental and behavioral healthcare has been blamed on Black people is the healthcare system's failure to provide substance use treatment and instead criminalize substance use. This is most visibly seen in the differential incarceration and treatment rates for substance use for Black compared with White Americans.

In 1986, as part of former President Ronald Reagan's "War on Drugs," the US Congress passed the Anti–Drug Abuse Act. The War on Drugs is sometimes referred to as the "War on Black People," as many of its policies were steered to criminalize activities that were more policed in Black communities. For example, under the Anti–Drug Abuse Act of 1986, and expanded in the 1988 Omnibus Anti–Drug Abuse Act, different penalties were attached to different types of cocaine usage, and as a first in US history, established mandatory incarceration sentencing for different quantities of cocaine. Crack cocaine was cheaper and more accessible to people with low incomes, who were disproportionately Black, while powder cocaine was more expensive and more prevalently used by affluent White people. Distribution of just 5 grams of crack carried a minimum sentence of 5 years in federal prison, while it would take distribution of 500 grams of powder to earn the same sentence—100 times the amount of crack cocaine. This 100:1 ratio for sentencing set up the false notion that crack and powder cocaine were differentially harmful, even though the US Sentencing Commission continued to show that crack and powder cocaine were not significantly different in their behavioral or physiological effects (Vagins and McCurdy 2006). Additionally, media propaganda at the time about the "devil drug" crack showed contrasting images of Black and Latine people living in the inner city as addicts and criminals, while White people were portrayed as victims (Santoro and Santoro 2018; Garske 2018).

Both the sentencing ratio and the images contributed to drug use being assigned as a moral and individual failure, rather than a medical issue. Black drug users were sentenced to federal prison, rather than being offered healthcare for addiction, resulting in disproportionate incarceration rates for Black people. In fact, the Anti–Drug Abuse Act of 1986 contributed to the quadrupling of the prison population between 1980 and 2000, two-thirds of which were charged of drug possession. This led to disproportionate incarceration of Black men and women. Despite Black and White people having similar rates of drug use, Black people are three times more likely to be incarcerated for drug possession (Nellis 2021)——contributing to family separations and ineligibility for social services for people who were already socioeconomically challenged (Vagins and McCurdy 2006).

Unsubstantiated claims about the differential health impacts of crack and powder cocaine were common myths used to support discriminatory laws. This included, for example, the myth that maternal crack usage created "crack babies," even though studies found that crack and powder cocaine had the same impact on fetal outcomes, or the myth that crack was more addictive than powder cocaine, which was also untrue. The shield of improving health was once again being used to reinforce and support discriminatory policies.

The impact of this 1986 law was finally addressed over twenty years later under former President Barack Obama's 2010 Fair Sentencing Act (American Civil Liberties Union 2010), which originally was written to completely eliminate the disparity in federal sentencing of crack and cocaine possession; however, in a capitulation to the Republican Senate Judiciary Committee members, the sentencing ratio was instead reduced from 100:1 to 18:1.

We are still undoing the harms caused by our criminalization of healthcare needs, while also fighting new policies that criminalize healthcare needs. Some of this same rhetoric has been used in the response to the opioid epidemic in the US (Bridges 2020), leading heroin use in Black communities to be criminalized while opioid-based drug addiction in White communities is medicalized.

The tactics and targets used to criminalize healthcare continue to be reproduced in minoritized populations in the US. In 2022, as Dr. Madina Agénor has documented in state-level policies around sexual and gender minority health(Agénor et al. 2021, 2022; Brown University Library n.d.), several states introduced bills criminalizing life-saving gender-affirming care for children and youth identifying as transgender (Rayasam 2022). Similarly, several states criminalize abortion care (Center for Reproductive Rights 2022). In contrast to the Anti–Drug Abuse Act that criminalized individuals possessing drugs, these bills often penalize healthcare providers who provide care or prohibit state-sponsored health insurance from providing treatments (Geggis 2023).

Conclusion

These examples of how the advancement of health and medical science has been used to oppress people are not intended to cause shame but, instead, are intended for reflection and consideration of how to be intentional about avoiding future insults and harm. These are not simply historical examples; these examples continue to bear fruit or emerge in our present-day society, and we are often unknowingly complicit in endorsing or reproducing them, sometimes due to the social norms of the day or because there are direct or indirect incentives or gains afforded to us. While pursuing scientific advancement in health and medicine can be of great benefit, consider the expense of what and to whom and whether that resonates with ethical principles and commitments to equity. We must reframe the narrative that we cannot truly have public health advancement or progress without equity—that is, there is no true progress unless its benefits are equitably shared.

References

Center for Reproductive Rights. 2022. "After Roe Fell: Abortion Laws by State." https://reproductiverights.org/maps/abortion-laws-by-state/.

Agénor M., C. Perkins, C. Stamoulis, et al. 2021. "Developing a Database of Structural Racism–Related State Laws for Health Equity Research and Practice in the United States." *Public Health Reports* 136 (4): 428-440. doi:10.1177/0033354920984168

Agénor, Madina, Ashley E. Pérez, Alexa L. Solazzo, Ariel L. Beccia, Mihail Samnaliev, Janson Wu, Brittany M. Charlton, and S. Bryn Austin. 2022. "Assessing Variations in Sexual Orientation- and Gender Identity-Related U.S. State Laws for Sexual and Gender Minority Health Research and Action, 1996-2016." *LGBT Health* 9 (3): 207–216.

American Civil Liberties Union. 2010. "President Obama Signs Bill Reducing Cocaine Sentencing Disparity." https://www.aclu.org/press-releases/president-obama-signs-bill-reducing-cocaine-sentencing-disparity.

Associated Press. 2022. "Philadelphia Apologizes for Experiments on Black Inmates." NPR, https://www.npr.org/2022/10/07/1127406363/philadelphia-apologizes-experiments-black-inmates.

Baptiste, Diana-Lyn, Nicole Caviness-Ashe, Nia Josiah, Yvonne Commodore-Mensah, Joyell Arscott, Patty R. Wilson, and Shaquita Starks. 2022. "Henrietta Lacks and America's Dark History of Research Involving African Americans." *Nursing Open* 9 (5): 2236.

Bassett, Mary T. 2016. "Beyond Berets: The Black Panthers as Health Activists." *American Journal of Public Health* 106 (10): 1741–1743.

Bigby, Michael E. 1999. "Acres of Skin: Human Experimentation at Holmesburg Prison." *Archives of Dermatology* 135 (4): 477–478.

Blackburn, Marsha. 2021. "Why Is Critical Race Theory Dangerous for Our Kids?" Marsha Blackburn. https://www.blackburn.senate.gov/2021/7/why-is-critical-race-theory-dangerous-for-our-kids.

Blain, Keisha N., and Tom Zoellner. 2020. "'Riots', 'Mobs', 'Chaos': The Establishment Always Frames Change as Dangerous." *The Guardian*. https://www.theguardian.com/commentisfree/2020/jun/10/protest-black-lives-matter-police-activism.

Boarding School Healing Project. 2011. *Reparations and American Indian Boarding Schools: A Critical Appraisal.* Boarding School Healing Project.

Bridges, Khiara M. 2020. "Race, Pregnancy, and the Opioid Epidemic: White Privilege and the Criminalization of Opioid Use During Pregnancy." *Harvard Law Review* 133 (3): 770–851.

Brown University Library. "Brown Digital Repository." n.d. Accessed February 7, 2024. https://repository.library.brown.edu/studio/.

Brown, Jalen, and Hannah Sarisohn. 2022. "Philadelphia Apologizes for History of Prison Experiments on Black Men, Hopes to Rectify Medical Mistrust within Community." CNN, https://www.cnn.com/2022/10/07/us/philadelphia-apologizes-prison-experiments-black-men-reaj/index.html.

Brown, Lawrence T. 2021. *The Black Butterfly: The Harmful Politics of Race and Space in America.* JHU Press.

Campbell, Kendall M., Irma Corral, Jhojana L. Infante Linares, and Dmitry Tumin. 2020. "Projected Estimates of African American Medical Graduates of Closed Historically Black Medical Schools." *JAMA Network Open* 3 (8): e2015220.

Cartwright, Samuel A. 1851. "Report on the Diseases and Physical Peculiarities of the Negro Race (1851)." In *The Nature of Difference: Sciences of Race in the United States from Jefferson to Genomics*, edited by Evelynn M. Hammonds and Rebecca M. Herzig, 67–86. MIT Press.

Chalfant, Morgan. 2021. "Biden Reverses Trump Order Barring Immigrants Who Cannot Afford Healthcare." The Hill. https://thehill.com/homenews/administration/553629-biden-revokes-trump-era-order-barring-immigrants-who-cannot-afford/.

Clauset, Aaron, Samuel Arbesman, and Daniel B. Larremore. 2015. "Systematic Inequality and Hierarchy in Faculty Hiring Networks." *Science Advances* 1 (1): e1400005.

Dean, Lorraine T., and Keon L. Gilbert. 2013. "Social Capital, Social Policy, and Health Disparities: A Legacy of Political Advocacy in African-American Communities." In *Global Perspectives on Social Capital and Health*, edited by Ichiro Kawachi, Soshi Takao, and S. V. Subramanian, 307–322. Springer New York.

Dean, Lorraine T., Amy Hillier, Hang Chau-Glendinning, S. V. Subramanian, David R. Williams, and Ichiro Kawachi. 2015. "Can You Party Your Way to Better Health? A Propensity Score Analysis of Block Parties and Health." *Social Science & Medicine* 138 (August): 201–209.

Doege, T. C. 1965. "Tuberculosis Mortality in the United States, 1900 to 1960." *JAMA* 192 (June): 1045–1048.

Duffy, Thomas P. 2011. "The Flexner Report: 100 Years Later." *Yale Journal of Biology and Medicine* 84 (3): 269–276.

Dula, Annette. 1994. "African American Suspicion of the Healthcare System Is Justified: What Do We Do About It?" *Cambridge Quarterly of Healthcare Ethics* 3 (3): 347–357.

Ferrieri, P., A. S. Dajani, and L. W. Wannamaker. 1973. "Benzathine Penicillin in the Prophylaxis of Streptococcal Skin Infections: A Pilot Study." *Journal of Pediatrics* 83 (4): 572–577.

Ferrieri, P., A. S. Dajani, and L. W. Wannamaker. 1974. "A Controlled Study of Penicillin Prophylaxis against Streptococcal Impetigo." *Journal of Infectious Diseases* 129 (4): 429–438.

Flexner, Abraham. 1910. *Medical Education in the United States and Canada: A Report to the Carnegie Foundation for the Advancement of Teaching*. Carnegie Foundation for the Advancement of Teaching. https://play.google.com/store/books/details?id=B4EfAAAAYAAJ.

Furlow, Bryant. 2020. "A Hospital's Secret Coronavirus Policy Separated Native American Mothers from Their Newborns." https://www.propublica.org/article/a-hospitals-secret-coronavirus-policy-separated-native-american-mothers-from-their-newborns.

Gamble, Vanessa Northington. 1995. *Making a Place for Ourselves: The Black Hospital Movement, 1920-1945*. Oxford University Press.

Gamble, V. N. 1997. "Under the Shadow of Tuskegee: African Americans and Health Care." *American Journal of Public Health* 87 (11): 1773–1778.

Garske, Caroline. 2018. "*Crack in the System: The Racially Motivated Intentions and Consequences of the Anti-Drug Abuse Act of 1986.*" University of Iowa. https://core.ac.uk/download/pdf/213512529.pdf.

Geggis, Anne. 2023. "Bill Criminalizing Gender-Affirming Treatment Advances." Florida Politics. https://floridapolitics.com/archives/594939-bill-criminalizing-gender-affirming-treatment-advances/.

Geller, Jeffrey. 2020. "Structural Racism in American Psychiatry and APA: Part 8." *Psychiatric News* 55 (20). https://doi.org/10.1176/appi.pn.2020.10b29.

Gilbert, Keon L., Yusuf Ransome, Lorraine T. Dean, Jerell DeCaille, and Ichiro Kawachi. 2022. "Social Capital, Black Social Mobility, and Health Disparities." *Annual Review of Public Health* 43: 173–191.

Goar, C. 2008. "Experiments in Black and White: Power and Privilege in Experimental Methodology." In *White Logic, White Methods: Racism and Methodology*, edited by Tukufu Zuberi and Eduardo Bonilla-Silva, 156. Rowman & Littlefield.

Hornblum, Allen M. 2013. *Acres of Skin: Human Experiments at Holmesburg Prison.* Routledge.

National Academy of Sciences, National Academy of Engineering, and Institute of Medicine. 2011. *Expanding Underrepresented Minority Participation: America's Science and Technology Talent at the Crossroads.* National Academies Press.

Jarvis, Edward. 1842. "Statistics of Insanity in the United States." *Boston Medical and Surgical Journal* 27 (7): 116–121.

Jones, David S., Scott H. Podolsky, Meghan Bannon Kerr, and Evelynn Hammonds. 2023. "Slavery and the Journal: Reckoning with History and Complicity." *New England Journal of Medicine* 389 (23): 2117–2123.

Kendi, I. X. 2016. *Stamped from the Beginning: The Definitive History of Racist Ideas in America.*" Hachette UK.

Krieger, N. 2000. "Epidemiology and Social Sciences: Towards a Critical Reengagement in the 21st Century." *Epidemiologic Reviews* 22 (1): 155–163.

Krishnan, Lakshmi, S. Michelle Ogunwole, and Lisa A. Cooper. 2020. "Historical Insights on Coronavirus Disease 2019 (COVID-19), the 1918 Influenza Pandemic, and Racial Disparities: Illuminating a Path Forward." *Annals of Internal Medicine* 173 (6): 474–481.

LaVeist, T. A., K. J. Nickerson, and J. V. Bowie. 2000. "Attitudes about Racism, Medical Mistrust, and Satisfaction with Care among African American and White Cardiac Patients." *Medical Care Research and Review* 57 (Suppl 1): 146–161.

Laws, Terri. 2021. "How Should We Respond to Racist Legacies in Health Professions Education Originating in the Flexner Report?" *AMA* 23 (3): E271–E275.

Lett, Elle, Dalí Adekunle, Patrick McMurray, Emmanuella Ngozi Asabor, Whitney Irie, Melissa A. Simon, Rachel Hardeman, and Monica R. McLemore. 2022. "Health

Equity Tourism: Ravaging the Justice Landscape." *Journal of Medical Systems* 46 (3): 17.

Loyola University Maryland. 2019. "1910: The Great Migration." The Baltimore Story. https://www.thebaltimorestory.org/history-1/blog-post-title-four-hc9z5.

Ly, Dan P. 2022. "Historical Trends in the Representativeness and Incomes of Black Physicians, 1900-2018." *Journal of General Internal Medicine* 37 (5): 1310–1312.

MacLure, Jennifer. 2021. "Unnatural Resources: The Colonial Logic of the Holmesburg Prison Experiments." *Journal of Medical Humanities* 42 (3): 423–433.

Miller, Lynn E., and Richard M. Weiss. 2012. "Revisiting Black Medical School Extinctions in the Flexner Era." *Journal of the History of Medicine and Allied Sciences* 67 (2): 217–243.

Morabia, Alfredo. 2016. "Unveiling the Black Panther Party Legacy to Public Health." *American Journal of Public Health* 106 (10): 1732–1733.

Morgan, Allison C., Nicholas LaBerge, Daniel B. Larremore, Mirta Galesic, Jennie E. Brand, and Aaron Clauset. 2022. "Socioeconomic Roots of Academic Faculty." *Nature Human Behaviour* 6 (12): 1625–1633.

Nellis, Ashley. 2021. "The Color of Justice: Racial and Ethnic Disparity in State Prisons." The Sentencing Project. https://www.sentencingproject.org/app/uploads/2022/08/The-Color-of-Justice-Racial-and-Ethnic-Disparity-in-State-Prisons.pdf.

Nuriddin, Ayah, Graham Mooney, and Alexandre I. R. White. 2020. "Reckoning with Histories of Medical Racism and Violence in the USA." *Lancet* 396 (10256): 949–951.

Pollard, Sam. 2012. "Jim Crow & Plessy v. Ferguson," *Slavery by Another Name* (movie). TPT National Productions in association with Two Dollars & A Dream.

Plessy v. Ferguson. 1896, 163 U.S. 537.

Power, Garrett. 1983. "Apartheid Baltimore Style: The Residential Segregation Ordinances of 1910-1913." *Maryland Law Review* 42 (2): 289.

Price, Gregory N., William Darity, and Rhonda V. Sharpe. 2020. "Did North Carolina Economically Breed-Out Blacks during Its Historical Eugenic Sterilization Campaign?" *American Review of Political Economy* 15 (1).

Rathbun, Lyon. 2001. "The Debate over Annexing Texas and the Emergence of Manifest Destiny." *Rhetoric and Public Affairs* 4 (3): 459–494.

Rayasam, Renuka. 2022. "The Transgender Care that States Are Banning, Explained." Politico. https://www.politico.com/newsletters/politico-nightly/2022/03/25/the-transgender-care-that-states-are-banning-explained-00020580.

Roberts, Samuel. 2003. "'Where Our Melanotic Citizens Predominate': Locating African Americans and Finding the 'Lung Block' in Tuberculosis Research in Baltimore, Maryland, 1880-1920." In *CrossRoutes, the Meanings of "Race" for the 21st Century*, edited by Paola Boi and Sabine Broeck, 91–112. LIT Verlag Münster.

Santoro, Taylor N., and Jonathan D. Santoro. 2018. "Racial Bias in the US Opioid Epidemic: A Review of the History of Systemic Bias and Implications for Care." *Cureus* 10 (12): e3733.

Shear, Michael D., and Miriam Jordan. 2019. "Trump Will Deny Immigrant Visas to Those Who Can't Pay for Health Care." *New York Times*, October 5. https://www.nytimes.com/2019/10/04/us/immigrant-visas-health-care.html.

Smith, Andrea. 2004. "Boarding School Abuses, Human Rights, and Reparations." *Social Justice* 31 (4 (98)): 89–102.

Solomon, Teshia G. Arambula, Rachel Rose Bobelu Starks, Agnes Attakai, Fatima Molina, Felina Cordova-Marks, Michelle Kahn-John, Chester L. Antone, Miguel Flores Jr, and Francisco Garcia. 2022. "The Generational Impact of Racism on Health: Voices from American Indian Communities." *Health Affairs* 41 (2): 281–288.

Sommers, Benjamin D., Anna L. Goldman, Robert J. Blendon, E. John Orav, and Arnold M. Epstein. 2019. "Medicaid Work Requirements: Results from the First Year in Arkansas." *New England Journal of Medicine* 381 (11): 1073–1082.

Staff Writer. 1918. "New Segregation Plan: Mayor Begins Work of Securing a Special Ordinance." *Baltimore Sun*, July 2.

Steinecke, Ann, and Charles Terrell. 2010. "Progress for Whose Future? The Impact of the Flexner Report on Medical Education for Racial and Ethnic Minority Physicians in the United States." *Academic Medicine* 85 (2): 236–245.

Sternberg, S. 2015. "Desegregation: The Hidden Legacy of Medicare." *U.S. News & World Report*.

Tennessee General Assembly. n.d. "HB0580/SB0623." https://wapp.capitol.tn.gov/apps/BillInfo/Default.aspx?BillNumber=SB0623.

Thomas, S. B., and S. C. Quinn. 1991. "The Tuskegee Syphilis Study, 1932 to 1972: Implications for HIV Education and AIDS Risk Education Programs in the Black Community." *American Journal of Public Health* 81 (11): 1498–1505.

The TRUTH Project. 2023. "Oshkigin Noojimo'iwe, Naǧi Waŋ P̣etu Uŋ Ihduwaṡ'ake He Oyate Kiŋ Zaniwiçaye Kte." https://mn.gov/indian-affairs/assets/full-report_tcm1193-572488.pdf.

US Bureau of the Census. 1975. *Historical Statistics of the United States, Colonial Times to 1970*. US Department of Commerce, Bureau of the Census.

Vagins, Deborah J., and Jesselyn McCurdy. 2006. *"Cracks in the System: Twenty Years of the Unjust Federal Crack Cocaine Law."* American Civil Liberties Union. https://www.aclu.org/documents/cracks-system-20-years-unjust-federal-crack-cocaine-law.

Vinokour, Maya. 2023. "Work Won't Set You Free." *Boston Globe*. https://www.bostonglobe.com/2023/08/07/opinion/florida-board-education-slavery-nazism/.

Williams, Heather Andrea. 2014. *American Slavery: A Very Short Introduction.* Oxford University Press.

Zinn, Howard. 2005. *A People's History of the United States.* HarperCollins.

Zuberi, Tukufu, and Eduardo Bonilla-Silva. 2008. *White Logic, White Methods: Racism and Methodology.* Rowman & Littlefield Publishers.

Chapter 12

Inclusive Classroom and Evaluation Activities

Deconstructing Privilege while Building Coalitions

Eric César Morales and Lorraine T. Dean

As a society, we are reaching a pivotal opportunity: we are better at understanding how the concept of privilege applies to every aspect of human civilization (from the classroom, hospital, and courtroom to where we work and live and with whom we interact in our social lives), but we still struggle with how to teach this complex concept in ways that are equally relevant to every racial, cultural, ethnic, or social class. Oftentimes, our approach to teaching privilege, ironically, focuses almost entirely on educating White students, with students of color, at best, left out of the discussion entirely or, at worst, used as cautionary tales to illustrate how bad things could be. When we teach White students why American society favors many of their attributes, we often run into numerous issues: the thought that successes might be the direct result of privilege leads some White students to deny the construct of privilege altogether, or the realization that the cards are stacked against students of color might discourage them and thus become a self-fulfilling prophecy. It can also lead to an unproductive practice of "ritualistic confessions" wherein White students are asked to identify how White privilege operates in their lives and if they are willing to repudiate that privilege, which of itself, can be unproductive and can overly focus attention on individual rather than structural elements that contribute to privilege (Lensmire et al. 2013). Further complicating matters is that there is more than one type of privilege, and when we focus on race, students miss out on learning how society responds to and reinforces the constellations of our identities.

To remedy these challenges, this chapter will offer practical illustrative exercises instructors can use to encourage all students to recognize the

Eric César Morales and Lorraine T. Dean, *Inclusive Classroom and Evaluation Activities*. In: *Power, Privilege, and Public Health in the United States*. Edited by: Lorraine T. Dean and Keilah A. Jacques, Oxford University Press. © Oxford University Press (2025). DOI: 10.1093/9780197760956.003.0012 complex social power dynamics that undergird human society. These constructive activities are designed to both teach about privilege and build coalitions, bringing everyone to solutions and sharing accountability for dismantling structures of privilege. As you tread into what can become a divisive territory, however, we offer a phrase of guidance: we must all become more comfortable with being uncomfortable. As we do so, we can prepare and reflect on how to use that discomfort to power us toward greater equity.

Evaluating and Designing Teaching Strategies on Privilege

In 1988, Peggy McIntosh attempted to verbalize her own experiences of being a White woman in a White world when she published the foundational article, "White Privilege: Unpacking the Invisible Knapsack" (McIntosh 1988). It is a powerful piece where she delineates numerous benefits resulting from her Whiteness that accompany her wherever she goes, and in the process, she asks us to reflect on our own invisible knapsacks of privilege. On the surface, creating our own lists of privileges might provide an opportunity to show gratitude, which studies show is good for our emotional well-being (Watkins et al. 2003), and pushing to have these conversations was a transformational moment, particularly for that time period. In practice, however, this article is designed for the education of White people, and subsequently, it was adapted into activities that harm people of color.

For example, "stepping into the circle" is perhaps one of the most recognizable activities to do so. For this activity, an instructor reads from a list of identifying characteristics or personal struggles to a group of students standing around a circle, and when a student hears an item that corresponds to their lives, they step into the circle and then step out. A similar and far more injurious activity is "the privilege walk," where people standing on a horizontal line step forward or backward, depending on whether aspects of their lives coincide with a list read by the instructor. Many of the prompts read by the instructors in these activities are pulled directly from McIntosh's article. For both activities, people who have suffered the most, usually students of color, are asked to visibly represent their adversities for the benefit of people whom society has already privileged—largely cis, able-bodied, upper-class, heterosexual, White men. Unfortunately, while it should go without saying that an instructor should not use one student's trauma as a teaching tool for another, these activities are central to almost all diversity training.

Peggy McIntosh most likely did not intend for her work to lead to these types of exercises, but examining how they fail can help us create more effective strategies. To do so, we must accept a few key principles:

- With every teaching activity on privilege, we must ask ourselves, "What do our most disadvantaged students have to gain?" If the answer is simply having others learn they are privileged, then we have succeeded only in perpetuating a system that centers those with privilege.
- The activities should go beyond simply showing privilege and move toward inviting conversation about how to navigate and dismantle privilege structures in the real world.
- We must refrain from the impulse of maintaining an academic distance from the subject matter. When we speak about privilege, our positionality matters, as we are intimately involving each group we move within and every aspect of our backgrounds.
- We must share that we do not have the answers and that we, like everyone else, are still trying to figure out how to operate in a world where we regularly alternate from being the beneficiaries to being the unfortunate recipients of inequities.
- We must validate the difficult feelings these conversations can bring up in our students. As long as they approach these topics with open minds, it is okay for them to feel uneasy, because the topic is messy.
- We must allow ourselves to sit in discomfort sometimes, for it provides us with an opportunity to reevaluate our own behaviors, inclinations, and biases. This includes acknowledging that no matter our intentions, we are not immune to perpetuating inequities.
- Finally, we must give ourselves grace and ask for it in turn, sharing the understanding that while we may stumble in this subject matter, it is okay to do so if we are committed to moving forward.

The following activities lay a foundation for understanding groups and how our association with a group provides privilege, preparing us to examine the topic in more depth. In many cases, these activities do not engage with Whiteness directly, nor should they. Far too often, our attempts to be more diverse fall into the refrain of centering Whiteness, often at the expense of people of color. For instance, anyone of color who has had to write a "commitment to diversity" essay knows how grueling this topic is, since institutions that usually ask for it tend to be predominantly White; in those circumstances, our attempts to exist in a space not designed for us should be seen as our commitment to diversity. In a similar vein, health or medical schools requiring "diversity essays" often prompt candidates to write about experiences where they learned something from people unlike themselves or to describe how they would handle hypothetical encounters with ethnicities different from themselves.[1] People of color going through the American education system, more likely than not, have primarily only had instructors of a different ethnic background, and those experiences have not always been positive—as can also be said about our experiences as medical patients. In the vein of offering constructive alternatives, a more insightful diversity statement would be for a person of color to write about an experience when someone from their background helped them understand what it's like to be the "diverse" individual moving in a White world.

The following activities are designed to build upon one another, successively deepening a student's understanding of privilege and taking them from a general knowledge of group formation to a holistic comprehension of the constantly shifting social structures we find ourselves in. As such, these activities are most effective when used periodically throughout the semester, which will allow for a fruitful examination of the construction of group identity, the contextual elements of identifying privilege, and the multifaceted ways that privilege manifests. Each section will include suggested readings and/or accessible video content as well as reflection questions to stimulate open-ended discussions among students, helping them draw unique connections between the concept of privilege and the realities of their daily lives. After each exercise, we also provide an analytical, first-person reflection on how the lesson plan has worked in our respective courses. Although this is a book about health, these activities may be adapted for use across a range of fields and disciplines.

Teaching Topic: Group Identity

Privilege has multiple permutations, as it can be expressed in terms of race, gender, sexuality, social class, ability, and more. Studies of intersectional privilege reveal the various ways these group associations influence each other and impact individual lives (Cech 2022; Case 2018), ultimately impacting the ease with which people find themselves in medical or health-related fields. Central to a nuanced understanding of privilege is the ability to grasp the formation and prioritization of group identity and welfare. This is because, at

---

[1] *This American Life* has a wonderful podcast about this, detailing an experience where a high school student, Mariya Karimjee, with Pakistani heritage ended up reading dozens of "diversity essays" written by her peers who described meeting Mariya: https://www.thisamericanlife.org/625/transcript.

its core, privilege comes from one's association with an empowered group. A strong activity to elicit this understanding is "the student's dilemma" (Table 12.1).

This activity is an adaptation of the prisoner's dilemma, which is perhaps one of the most famous examples of game theory—a blend of psychology and math that examines strategic and logical decision-making between rational adults. The prisoner's dilemma outlines a scenario where police attempt to have one of two accused criminals turn on their friend by offering them leniency or certain privileges, such as immunity from prosecution. The question at the center of this dilemma is simple: Can we trust others to place the good of the whole over their individual advancement?

The prisoner's dilemma has been applied to a variety of real-life situations throughout history, from the Cold War (Plous 1993) to the Paris Climate Accords (Gillani 2022); the countries' respective decisions become a synecdoche, representing the will of the whole, with all members benefiting or suffering due to that decision, whether or not they agree with it. When adapting the prisoner's dilemma to a classroom setting, the goals are for students to see how easily groups form, how self-interests become prioritized, and how even people who might want to distance themselves from the choices of the group still benefit or are harmed by those choices. Examining this group association then provides insight into the underpinnings of larger social issues that drive health inequities, like income inequality, poverty, police brutality, and structural racism.

A quick disclaimer: the following activity is most effective when conducted on the first day of class, and it is a much more interesting and less anxiety-inducing icebreaker than the standard "Tell us your name and one thing you find interesting about yourself." After all, let's be honest, most people are so worried about saying something interesting that almost no one is paying any real attention until after they themselves speak.

Classroom Analysis

Attribution: Eric César Morales

The beauty of the student's dilemma activity is that it does not matter if students make it through all three rounds, as every stage of the process repeatedly encourages students to think about their identity as it relates to different spheres: the individual, the small group, and the larger whole. For years, I conducted this activity with each one of my undergraduate courses, and while

Table 12.1 The Student's Dilemma

	Resources Needed: Index cards, writing utensils, timer	**Recommended class size: 16–40**
Activity Description	For this activity, divide students into groups of four, with the only caveat being that members of the group must not know each other beforehand. Once students are in these small groups, have them introduce themselves to each other and then find three things all members of the group have in common, the more specific the better. Examples can be hobbies, being the oldest child, favorite television shows, or even the part of town they live in. The more unique the connection drawn, the more effective and cohesive the group becomes. Once students find the three commonalities, have them create a group name based on one of them and have each group share these commonalities and the resulting names with the rest of the class.	
	At this stage, inform the entire class that there will be an opportunity for every student to earn five extra credit points[b] or for one group to earn twenty extra credit points while everyone else gets nothing. For everyone to earn the five points, the whole class must pass three rounds in which they have to unanimously agree to share the points. If one group elects to earn more points for themselves, the rest of the class gets nothing. The rules are as follows:	

continued

Table 12.1 *continued*

	Resources Needed: Index cards, writing utensils, timer	Recommended class size: 16–40
Round 1	1. Give each group an index card. Instruct them to draw a line down the middle of it with their group name written on one side of the line and the word "class" written on the other.	
	2. Give the class sixty seconds in which each group can deliberate among themselves on whether they want the class to potentially share five points by advancing to the next round or if they want each member in their individual team to earn ten points and end the game on this round. Groups are not allowed to talk to other groups.	
	3. At the end of the sixty seconds, instruct the groups to either circle their group name or the word "class." Make it clear that they cannot circle until the end of the sixty-second deliberation. Students should then hand the card to the instructor, who is standing in the middle of the room.	
	4. If each group chooses "class," then everyone advances to the next round. But the first group to hand the instructor a card with their group name circled, wins ten extra credit points, while the rest of the class gets nothing. a. If a group wins this round, ask the group why they chose to do so, and then advance to the lightning round.	
Round 2	5. Repeat steps 1–4, but the groups only have 45 seconds to deliberate, and the first group to hand a card with their group name circled gets 15 extra credit points.	
Round 3	6. Repeat steps 1–4, but the groups only have 30 seconds to deliberate, and the first group to hand a card with their group name circled gets 20 extra credit points.	
	7. If each group circled "class" then everyone wins and the game ends.	

Lightning round

To be played only if a group choses themselves over the class. In this round, each student from the winning group has an opportunity to win thirty points instead of twenty, but if they choose to do so, their other group members get nothing.

8. Give each member of the winning group an index card. Instruct them to draw a line down the middle, like before, but this time, have them write their name on one side and their group's on the other.

9. Instruct each student to stand in a different corner of the room, where they cannot see their team members, and give them twenty seconds to deliberate alone on whether they want to win thirty points for themselves or for each group member to keep twenty points.

10. At the end of the twenty seconds, have them circle either their name or the group name and hand the card to the instructor in the center of the room. As before, only the first person to hand in their circled name gets the points.

Suggested readings/videos

Noyes, Dory. 2010. "Groups." In *Eight Words for the Study of Expressive Culture*, edited by Burt Feintuch. University of Illinois Press. *Mean Girls*, 2004. Timestamp 9:05 to 11:55.

Discussion questions

- How do people form groups?
- What methods do groups use to maintain a connective thread between the members?
- How do groups go about adding new members?
- How do groups prioritize their own members above others?

---

[a]For this type of activity, we recommend offering extra credit rather than make it an actual assignment. This removes any grade anxiety students might have and allows them to behave more freely. Additionally, to avoid providing too many extra credit opportunities in a class, we recommend capping the amount of extra credit a student can earn, such as 30 to 35 points out of a 1,000-point scale.

[b]I suspect that other groups overheard this discussion, which led to the class actually sharing the points, so in the future, I made sure that groups deliberated among themselves quietly.

students always had fun with it, groups rarely made it past the second round. When it came time to ask students why they chose the options they did, the classroom conversations that took place were always insightful. In fact, they have fundamentally shaped the way I see the world.

The first class I used this activity with became one of the most noteworthy instances. The connective thread between the winning group members was that they were studying sociology, so they named themselves "The Sociologists." When I asked them why they chose to circle their own group name on the second round instead of share with the class, they responded, and I paraphrase, "We're learning that humans tend to operate in their best interests, so we wanted to get the points first because if we didn't, we knew someone else would beat us to it." Yet, when it came time to turn on other members of the group, no one did. When I asked why, they said, and I paraphrase, "I don't want the whole class to hate me. I still need some friends."

Every class was different in notable ways. Sometimes, there would be multiple groups who would want to sell out the class in the first round. Sometimes, it would be the third. Usually, when a group chose themselves, in their deliberations, there would be one group member loudly pushing for that option, and the rest of the members would fall in line. At times, one group member would make the decision alone to circle the group name, but everyone else still benefited from the action. In one notable deviation, the only instance where the whole class shared the points, one student kept insisting that they needed to put their group's interests over the class because if they didn't, another group would. In each round, she was countered by a single group member who would loudly exclaim, and I do not paraphrase, "I don't care if they do. Let them. I have one rule in life: Don't be shitty!"[2]

For this activity, I would not tend to ask too many questions of the class on the day of the activity, and I would like to say it's to let the students sit in thought. In reality, this activity generates so much excitement and is so novel that students often need a bit of distance before they evaluate what transpired and why they pushed for certain choices. Conversations about group identity, group formation, and the privilege that comes when one group is allowed to prioritize themselves over the good of the larger whole can be disconcerting, especially when the students are the ones making the decisions

---

[2] For this type of activity, it's best to offer extra credit rather than make it an actual assignment. This removes any grade anxiety students might have and allows them to behave more freely. Additionally, to avoid providing too many extra credit opportunities in a class,; we recommend capping the amount of extra credit a student can earn, such as 30–35 points out of a 1,000-point scale.

that shape the outcomes for the class. Besides, having some time before getting into a thorough discussion would also allow me to reflect on the events that transpired.

I would often revisit this activity, discussing it at different points in a semester. For instance, in a midterm exam, I would include an extra credit question where students are invited to reflect on the experience, and those were some of the richest responses I ever received. Students would share how surprised they were to create connections with group members so different from themselves and that the friends they made that day stayed close to them throughout the semester. Some would reflect on feeling bad that they pushed to be selfish or that they were surprised that most of the class wanted to share points and how it only took one person, unchecked by other members of their group, to change the outcome of the class. Ultimately, the realization I came away with was that the way we see the people around us dictates how we behave in the world. If we see others as naturally good, then we naturally want to be good. If we think everyone has their own selfish angle, then we may attempt to always get the upper hand. We reflect what we perceive in others.

Teaching Topic: The Privilege/Adversity Paradigm

One way we can more easily move forward with discussions around the concept of privilege is by teaching it as two separate theories: the privilege/adversity paradigm allows students to see that individual traits can be both positive and negative, depending on context, and colonizer alignment privilege guides us to understand how certain groups have created particular contexts to favor themselves (Morales 2020). This approach allows us to first focus on the importance of context in conceptions of privilege and then move on to how society creates and maintains a context that favors the colonizers of an area.

A strong activity to teach the privilege/adversity paradigm is the "This versus That Challenge" (Table 12.2). The inspiration for this activity comes from TikTok and YouTube personality Peet Montzingo, who regularly creates compelling content that features his family, all of whom have dwarfism except for him. At 6 feet 2 inches, he towers over his siblings and parents, and much of his content focuses on providing insights into what it was like growing up tall in a family of little people, often wishing he could be a little person as well. Rather than seeing being of above-average height as a blessing, he routinely comments on his childhood wish that he could have had more in common with

Table 12.2 "This versus That" Challenge

	Resources needed: Video/audio projector, paper, pencils	**Recommended class size:** Any size
Activity description	In this activity, the goal is to have students understand the important and shifting nature of context, so students are encouraged to see the benefits and drawbacks of their different traits. To avoid potential arguments, this activity should not directly take into consideration more polarizing concepts of race, gender, sexuality, weight, or social class.	
	Begin by introducing the class to Peet and Vicki Montzingo's social media presence—many students may already know them—and feel free to share a few of their videos to give students more background information. For instance, there are a pair of videos that, when juxtaposed, provide wonderful and contrasting perspectives on what it's like to be in a home entirely designed for people under 5 feet tall. In one video, Peet's tall friends visit Vicki's household and leave with hurt backs after spending so much time leaning over, and in the other, one of Peet's friends, who also has dwarfism, enters Vicki's home for the first time only to be elated due to finally being in a space designed for people of his stature. After students become more familiar with the material, play the first video from Peet Montzingo's series "Short vs Tall Challenge."	
Round 1: Short versus Tall	1. Separate students into groups of four, and encourage them to create new groups with classmates they have not partnered with before. Inform groups that they will come up with their own short versus tall scenarios.	
	2. Have each group take out a piece of paper and draw three columns. In the first column, have them write the word "context," in the second, "short," and in the third, "tall."	
	3. Give students 5–7 minutes to come up with four real-life contexts where someone's height matters:	
	a. Two of the scenarios must give preference to being short.	
	b. Two of the scenarios must give preference to being tall.	
	4. Have students share their findings with the class.	

Round 2: Introvert versus Extrovert	5. Repeat steps 1–4, but substitute the parameters.
Round 3: choose your own	6. Instruct students to see if they can come up with their own ideas for traits they want to juxtapose. Avoid selecting anything, however, that can be polarizing unless you trust in your ability to guide students through that terrain. If you would prefer to not come up with your own, another possible example is to have students examine being bilingual or the types of neurodivergence that are relatively recently being examined as having evolutionary advantages, such as ADHD (Reiss et al. 2022).
Suggested videos	"When My Tall Friends Come Over." https://www.youtube.com/shorts/w1lAd2sdwOE. "When Another Short Person Comes Over." https://www.youtube.com/shorts/M7fLUgpx1Pg. "Short vs Tall Challenge." https://www.youtube.com/shorts/1NSgK11RR-E. "Short vs Tall Challenge 2." https://www.youtube.com/shorts/sRMlfwT5cMw.
Discussion questions	• How often do we find ourselves in different contexts? • How do we know when we enter into a different context? • Why and how do we adjust to these contexts?

the people he loves and share life from their perspectives. His videos, in turn, celebrate his family, highlighting their wonderful personalities, particularly his charming mother, Vicki Montzingo, while also touching on important aspects of accessibility and general respect. In doing so, he shows that there is a lot to appreciate about life, no matter our differences. In November 2022, he published a children's picture book, *Little Imperfections: A Tall Tale of Growing Up Different*, to provide a space for everyone who doesn't feel like they fit into their families or communities and to also celebrate all the things that make us different.

One particularly entertaining and poignant series of videos he created is called "Short vs Tall Challenge," where he and his mother, Vicki, engage in numerous day-to-day activities, some of which advantage him and others, Vicki, based purely on height. This content provides the perfect foray into exploring the Privilege/Adversity Paradigm, as they are informative, accessible, and endearing, revealing how context impacts privilege.

Classroom Analysis

Attribution: Eric César Morales

The This versus That activity turns the table on students, challenging the notion that there is an ideal trait to have and, instead, encouraging everyone to find value in every aspect of themselves. In holding these exercises, what I did not expect was the amount of catharsis that students would feel when we explored the complexity of traits they happened to identify with. For instance, tall students would express so much vindication at having people acknowledge that there could be downsides to being above-average height, and this would genuinely be a shock to many other students. Conversely, discussions on the benefits of neurodivergence would often leave people feeling empowered. Rather than see themselves as having a condition that needed to be treated, they started to see their diagnoses as a normal variation of the state of being human. Sometimes, students with neurodivergence already had this perspective, and they were happy that someone else was doing the work of seeing their unique traits as potentially positive.

At no point in this exercise is a student requested to volunteer perspectives on traits they identify with, so when they do speak up, it always feels lighter. Since students can choose if and when to disclose, they do so when they feel safe. Their words then become a wonderful flourish, an adornment to the content of the discussion rather than the central focus.

Teaching Topic: Building Coalitions

The previous activity (Table 12.2) implicitly showed that we live in a hetero-topic society, where worlds exist next to and within other worlds (Foucault 1966). As privilege is connected to group identities, we can thus approach privilege as also existing in a heterotopia. Whenever we step into a new con-text, the privileges and advantages of our unique identity crystallization shift as well. This understanding is central to exploring colonizer alignment priv-ilege, which allows for "the various seen and unseen ways in which a person derives privilege due to how aligned they are with the colonizers of an area" (Morales 2020). With the next activity (Table 12.3), our goal is to help students "try on" being along the spectrum of power and privilege and use collective action to reflect on and address it.

Classroom Analysis

Attribution: Lorraine T. Dean

Every course cycle, the Privilege Adjustment Experiment (Table 12.3) is among the most eye-opening course activities. The first time I conducted this assignment, I did not know what to expect or how it would turn out. The biggest surprise was the astonishment that I would hear from students. Many didn't even notice that the experiment had happened, especially those who had received positive points. The first year it was conducted, one stu-dent exclaimed, "Why are the points randomly assigned—they should at least be based on *something*!" To which I replied, "You were randomly assigned into your social class; you did not choose the family you were born into. Randomly assigning points mimics the real experience of how unearned priv-ilege works." Another student, a White male, admitted that he hadn't noticed that he had received negative points and had just assumed that he had done very poorly on the assignment. To that, I explained, "That's the experience of *internalized discrimination*, the assumption that there is something inher-ently wrong with you or your work because of what society has arbitrarily assigned, not because of your actions."

The most interesting part of this activity is that each year brings some-thing unexpected, especially since each course must design its own solution to the privilege adjustment problem. That first year, some students, in protest, threatened to report me directly to the dean as being unethical but quickly abandoned that once they saw the value in the assignment. Later, that same

Table 12.3 The Privilege Adjustment Experiment

	Resources Needed: An existing graded assignment	Recommended class size: Any size
Activity description	We recommend doing this activity discreetly—that is, do not tell students up front that they are taking part in it. The activity adjusts the points in one of the other graded assignments offered in the course and requires that the students work together to devise solutions for overcoming this random point allocation. By having the activity impact the students' grades, it has real-life consequences for students, so they have a more authentic alignment experience.	
	At some point during the semester, preferably midsemester, take any one assignment, exam, or activity where students can physically see or track their grade. This can also be done on an online grade-tracking system where you add an additional column for an assignment that was never included in the syllabus. Using a random number generator, assign each student a meaningful point value for your course, such as −5 to +5 points. This must be completely random. Then discreetly list the change as "PA" (for Privilege Adjustment) on the assignment.	
	Once a student vocalizes that they observed the change, open a classroom discussion on the random point allocation. Explain that each person in the course was randomly assigned a negative or positive point value to mimic how people are born into a society with greater or fewer "privilege points," which advantage some people and disadvantage others. Let the class know that the points have real grade implications and that this is an opportunity for them to build coalitions to address privilege. Their goal, by the end of the semester, is to present a collectively agreed-upon solution to the professor that addresses the privilege gradient that was created. If they choose to do nothing, or cannot agree on a solution or set of solutions, the points stay as-is, impacting their official grades.	
	A few caveats: students cannot cancel the activity and simply ask that all points be reverted; this activity reflects society, and the real-world aspects of privilege that impact us from birth are not so easily negated. Additionally, students may not use threats, force, or intimidation tactics.[a] Lastly, to preserve the activity's value for future classes, advise students to not share the activity with anyone outside the course, even after the end of the semester.	
Suggested reading	Fisher, Roger, William L. Ury, and Bruce Patton. 2011. *Getting to Yes: Negotiating Agreement Without Giving In*. Penguin.	

Table 12.3 *continued*

	Resources Needed: An existing graded assignment	Recommended class size: Any size
Discussion questions	• How does it feel to have received positive or negative points? • As a classroom, how can you come together to address this unequal system? • Does dismantling systems of privilege require one group to give up something to benefit another? • What arguments or incentives can you use to bring people into constructive discussion about privilege?	

[a]This activity is focused on the need to find diplomatic solutions. This is, however, markedly different from the arc of US history, where some advancements in civil rights and human rights have only come about due to the threat of violence. In Howard Zinn's book, *A People's History of the United States*, he outlines how advancements in women's rights, Black civil rights, and workers' rights were often due to the threat of boycott or civil unrest with damage to physical property or harm to people.

group of students decided to end the experiment by asking for reparations: that is, for the instructor to fill back in some of the points to the people receiving negative points while leaving those with positive points intact. Another year, students decided to donate a portion of points to other students and floated having those who received positive points do one of three extra credit assignments and donate the additional points to the students who received negative points. And yet another year, the students could not come to a collective solution by the end of the course, and the points stood as-is: no solution was offered, and those who lost points simply had to make up for it by performing harder in other assignments (similar to the real world!) or complete extra credit work.

As students designed solutions, it was interesting to watch how quickly the privileged students openly admitted that they had no motivation or incentive to do or change anything. In these instances, the students with negative points had the onus to cajole the others into discussion or action, which sometimes failed. The difficulty of creating successful coalitions in a small class among students, many of whom are friends, then provided a meaningful springboard into discussions on the uphill battle of dismantling structures of privilege in our wider society, which is far more diverse and inequitable.

Final Notes

The most effective lessons do not focus on teaching privilege. Rather, they prioritize teaching students how power structures are created, adapted, maintained, and upended, with the dynamics being capable of being seen in small class groups as well as larger international situations. Theories like colonizer alignment privilege attempt to get that message across—that privilege is a result of those structures, not of someone's physical or social characteristics. When students have that understanding, they can better value the power of coalitions and can be more prepared to engage with people across social and class divides.

Earlier in the chapter, we stated that "privilege comes from one's association with an empowered group," but the corollary to that statement is also true: that privilege is undone when multiple groups form meaningful, mutually beneficial coalitions. Thus, only when we work together for a common good do we begin to unravel the power structures imposed upon us.

How to effectively get this message across is an ongoing process of self-reflection and learning for all of us. No matter how long we sit with the subject, there will always be more space to grow. And grow we must. We hope that these lessons provide a spark, the beginnings of a new approach to teaching privilege where instructors like yourself design activities focused on bringing students together in conversation, helping them see the power held within each of their classmates, and guiding them to find a resonance, one that leads to greater harmony for us all.

References

Case, Kim A. 2018. "White Practitioners in Therapeutic Ally-Ance: An Intersectional Privilege Awareness Training Model." In *Whiteness and White Privilege in Psychotherapy* edited by Andrea L. Dottolo, Ellyn Kaschak, 97–112. Routledge.

Cech, Erin A. 2022. "The Intersectional Privilege of White Able-Bodied Heterosexual Men in STEM." *Science Advances* 8 (24): eabo1558.

Foucault, Michel. 1973. *The Order of Things*. New York: Vintage.

Gillani, Dayyab. 2022. "Climate Change and Political Letdown: Understanding Environmental Degradation through the Prisoner's Dilemma." *Journal of Political Studies* 29: 65.

Lensmire, Timothy, Shannon McManimon, Jessica Dockter Tierney, Mary Lee-Nichols, Zachary Casey, Audrey Lensmire, and Bryan Davis. 2013. "McIntosh as Synecdoche: How Teacher Education's Focus on White Privilege Undermines Antiracism." *Harvard Educational Review* 83 (3): 410–431.

McIntosh, P. 1988. "White Privilege and Male Privilege: A Personal Account of Coming to See Correspondences through Work in Women's Studies." Working paper no. 189. Wellesley Centers for Women. http://www.nationalseedproject.org/

images/documents/White_Privilege_and_Male_Privilege_Personal_Account-Peggy_McIntosh.pdf.

Morales, Eric César. 2020. "Building Racial Coalitions: Limitations and New Directions to Teaching 'White Privilege.'" *Race and Pedagogy Journal: Teaching and Learning for Justice* 4 (3): 3.

Plous, S. 1993. "The Nuclear Arms Race: Prisoner's Dilemma or Perceptual Dilemma?" *Journal of Peace Research* 30 (2): 163–179.

Reiss, Michael, Annie Swanepoel, John Launer, Graham Music, and Bernadette Wren. 2022. "Evolutionary Perspectives on Neurodevelopmental Disorders." In *Evolutionary Psychiatry: Current Perspectives on Evolution and Mental Health*, edited by Riadh Abed and Paul St John-Smith, 228–243. Cambridge, UK: Cambridge University Press.

Watkins, Philip C., Kathrane Woodward, Tamara Stone, and Russell L. Kolts. 2003. "Gratitude and Happiness: Development of a Measure of Gratitude, and Relationships with Subjective Well-being." *Social Behavior and Personality* 31 (5): 431–451.

Index